AF344382

The Inflammatory Bowel Disease Yearbook 2003

Remedica State of the Art series
ISSN 1472-4626

Also available
The Handbook of Diabetes Mellitus and Cardiovascular Disease
Kidney Transplantation
Management of Aterosclerotic Carotid Disease
Management of Peripheral Arterial Disease
Multiple Myeloma
Rheumatoid Arthritis
Viral Co-infections in HIV: Impact and Management

Published by Remedica Publishing Limited
32–38 Osnaburgh Street, London, NW1 3ND, UK

Tel: +44 20 7388 7677
Fax: +44 20 7388 7457
Email: books@remedica.com
www.remedica.com

Publisher: Andrew Ward
In-house editors: Emma Hawkridge & Cath Harris

© 2003 Remedica Publishing Limited

All rights reserved. No part of this publication may be reproduced, stored
in a retrieval system or transmitted in any form or by any means, electronic,
mechanical, photocopying, recording or otherwise, without the prior permission
of the publisher.

ISBN 1 901346 57 9
British Library Cataloguing-in Publication Data
A catalogue record for this book is available from the British Library

The Inflammatory Bowel Disease Yearbook 2003

Charles Bernstein, Editor

Professor
Inflammatory Bowel Disease Clinical and Research Center
John Buhler Research Centre
804F-715 McDermot Avenue
Winnipeg, MB, R3E 3P4
Canada

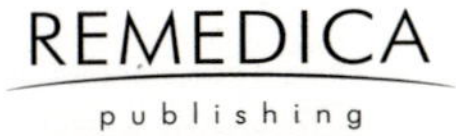

LONDON • CHICAGO

Contributors

Steven R Brant
Associate Professor of Medicine, Meyerhoff Inflammatory
Bowel Disease Center, Gastroenterology Division,
Department of Medicine, The Johns Hopkins University
School of Medicine, Baltimore, MD 21231, USA

Jean-Frédéric Colombel
Service des Maladies de l'Appareil Digestif et de la Nutrition,
INSERM, EPI 01/14, CHRU, Lille, France

Patrick Duthilleul
Département d'Hématologie-Immunologie-Cytogénétique,
CH Valenciennes, France

David G Forcione
Clinical and Research Fellow, Harvard Medical School;
Clinical Fellow in Medicine, Gastrointestinal Unit,
Massachusetts General Hospital, Boston, MA 02114, USA

Christoph Gasche
Associate Professor of Medicine, Medical University of Vienna;
Department of Medicine 4, Division of Gastroenterology,
General Hospital Vienna, Austria

Toshihiko Okazaki
Research Fellow, Meyerhoff Inflammatory Bowel Disease Center,
Gastroenterology Division, Department of Medicine,
The Johns Hopkins University School of Medicine
Baltimore, MD 21231, USA

Daniel Poulain
Laboratoire de Mycologie Fondamentale et Appliquée, INSERM,
EMI 99-15, CHRU et Faculté de Médecine, Lille, France

Dominique Reumaux
Département d'Hématologie-Immunologie-Cytogénétique,
CH Valenciennes, France

Bruce E Sands
Assistant Professor of Medicine, Harvard Medical School;
Assistant Physician, Gastrointestinal Unit, Massachusetts
General Hospital, Boston, MA 02114, USA

Boualem Sendid
Laboratoire de Mycologie Fondamentale et Appliquée, INSERM,
EMI 99-15, CHRU et Faculté de Médecine, Lille, France

Fergus Shanahan
Professor of Medicine, Department of Medicine,
University College Cork, National University of Ireland,
Clinical Science Building, Cork University Hospital, Ireland

A Hillary Steinhart
Associate Professor of Medicine, Universitiy of Toronto,
Room 445, Mount Sinai Hospital, 600 University Avenue,
Toronto, ON, M5G 1X5, Canada

Karl Turetschek
Associate Professor of Radiology, Department of Radiology,
Medical University Vienna and General Hospital Vienna, Austria

Preface

From a population health point of view, inflammatory bowel disease (IBD) is an increasing problem, for which novel approaches in diagnostics and therapeutics are rapidly evolving. IBD has also emerged as an important example of a complex chronic inflammatory disease where genetics, environmental risk factors, and individual phenotypic expression of disease interplay to establish patterns of disease and potential disease etiologies. The recent description of a gene specific for Crohn's disease (*NOD2*), the exploration of the role of microbes in disease causation, and the harnessing of microbes therapeutically (such as with probiotics) have facilitated the emergence of IBD as an important model amongst the chronic inflammatory diseases.

In a rapidly changing scientific environment, it is imperative for scientists and clinicians to have access to up-to-date reviews in the emerging areas of IBD therapy. Within this *IBD Yearbook*, we have assembled an international roster of clinician scientists to analyze and summarize very recent developments in six key areas of IBD.

Hillary Steinhart of the University of Toronto has reviewed conventional therapy (corticosteroids, 5-aminosalicylates, and antibiotics) in the context of the latest available information. These agents will continue to be used by clinicians in the foreseeable future.

David Forcione and Bruce Sands of Harvard Medical School have provided a concise update on novel biologic therapies in IBD. Their chapter provides the reader with insight into the use of available biologics as well as information on agents currently under study – some of which may soon be available for use.

Jean-Frederic Colombel and colleagues of the CHRU in Lille have reviewed state of the art data regarding serodiagnostics in IBD. Serum antibody tests are emerging as potentially key clinical diagnostic tools, and may also serve to enhance insights into disease pathogenesis.

Steven Brant and Toshihiko Okazaki of the Johns Hopkins University School of Medicine, Meyerhoff IBD Genetics Lab have summarized the myriad of IBD-specific genetic data, and in particular collated the data regarding *NOD2* and its associations with specific patterns of disease. Dr Brant and Dr Okazaki have also outlined potential IBD-related genes to be watched in the upcoming year.

Karl Turetschek of the Department of Radiology and Christoph Gasche of the Department of Medicine at the Medical University of Vienna have reviewed current approaches to imaging in IBD. Although some of the techniques may not be available in all community practices, most are available at major referral centers. These highlight the emergence of techniques that have potentially better resolution and diagnostic capability (such as helical CT enteroclysis) than more traditional imaging methods, or are minimally invasive (eg, capsule endoscopy).

Finally, Fergus Shanahan of the University College Cork, National University of Ireland has reviewed the emerging field of probiotics as a therapeutic tool in IBD. His chapter highlights the rationale for considering probiotic therapy in IBD, and summarizes the science of probiotic administration.

These chapters, written by internationally recognized leaders in IBD and their respective areas of research, have been assembled in this *IBD Yearbook*. For readers, it will provide a basis for interpreting the scientific literature that will be forthcoming in 2003 and beyond.

Charles Bernstein
John Buhler Research Centre

Contents

1

Conventional therapy

A Hillary Steinhart

Introduction

In recent years, there have been dramatic changes in the therapeutics of inflammatory bowel disease (IBD), and Crohn's disease (CD) in particular. This has been evidenced by the introduction of new biological therapies into the marketplace, ongoing studies of other biological therapies, growing interest in probiotics, and increasing use of immunomodulatory therapy.

Despite the introduction of new biological therapy into the therapeutic armamentarium, and the promise it holds for safe and effective treatment of IBD, research continues into the use of more "conventional" therapeutic agents. These include glucocorticoids, antibiotics, 5-aminosalicylic acid and its derivatives, and immunomodulatory drugs such as cyclosporine and azathioprine. This chapter discusses these agents and their appropriate place in the treatment of patients with ulcerative colitis (UC) and CD.

Glucocorticoids

Pharmacotherapy

The glucocorticoids remain the most consistently effective class of therapy for reducing the symptoms of IBD and for rapidly inducing clinical remission [1]. However, frequent use of glucocorticoids has generally been avoided or minimized by physicians and patients due to the significant potential for adverse effects such as weight gain, moon facies, mood disturbances, hypertension, diabetes, osteoporosis, and avascular necrosis to name but a few [2].

There has been considerable interest in the use of synthetic glucocorticoids, for example budesonide, a topically active glucocorticoid that undergoes high first-pass metabolism to form inactive metabolites in the liver. As a result, it has a more favorable side-effect profile compared with systemic glucocorticoids [3].

Budesonide has been formulated for use in the treatment of IBD in two different controlled-release formats (Entocort controlled ileal release [CIR] capsules, AstraZeneca; Budenofalk, Dr Falk, Pharma GmBH) that are designed to release the drug into the distal small bowel and colon. However, neither format has been specifically designed to release a significant portion of the drug beyond the proximal portion of the colon and, therefore, neither has been studied in UC. Most studies in CD have used the Entocort forumulation of budesonide, and this is the formulation that is currently available in North America.

An attempt was made to create a budesonide formulation designed specifically for colonic release. However, a study of this preparation in UC found that budesonide was not as effective as prednisolone, particularly with respect to control of inflammation in the more distal portions of the colon [4]. Although the study did show some promise, with reduction in inflammation on the right side of the colon, this formulation was not further developed and, as a result, most of the interest in orally administered budesonide has surrounded its potential for use in CD.

A desirable property of budesonide is its ability to be administered as a once daily dose rather than as multiple daily doses. The resulting efficacy is at least as good, if not better, than multiple daily dosing [5,6]. In healthy volunteers, it has been shown that the systemic absorption of Entocort CIR is 10%–13%, and is independent of the fasting or fed state [7].

Although the incidence of glucocorticoid-associated adverse events is lower with budesonide than with conventional glucocorticoids [3], it is still possible to detect measurable effects of budesonide on the hypothalamic–pituitary–adrenal axis by reductions in mean morning serum cortisol levels and corticotropin-stimulated cortisol levels [8]. Although this generally produces no clinical symptoms, it may be important in patients during periods of stress, eg, surgery.

Clinical trials

Initial studies of Entocort CIR demonstrated remission rates of 51%–69% in patients with ileal or ileocecal CD who received 9 mg budesonide daily over an 8-week study period [3,5,8,9]. However, more recent controlled trials have not found remission rates within the same range (see **Table 1**) [10,11].

Tremaine et al. carried out a multicenter, placebo-controlled trial of Entocort CIR in patients with CD of the ileum alone, or of the ileum and ascending colon [11]. The patients were given 9 mg budesonide daily as one or two divided doses. This study found remission rates of 48% and 53% in the one- and two-dose groups, respectively. Statistically, these remission rates were not significantly different from that observed in the placebo-treated patients (33%). The investigators argued that the lack of statistical significance was due to the higher than expected placebo rate, and that the remission rates observed in the budesonide-treated patients were not significantly different from those observed in previous studies of budesonide.

Steinhart et al. investigated combined budesonide and antibiotic therapy in patients with CD of the terminal ileum, with or without involvement of the ascending colon [10]. In this study, patients (N = 134) were randomized to receive oral ciprofloxacin and metronidazole, both 500 mg twice daily, or placebo for 8 weeks. All patients received budesonide (Entocort CIR), 9 mg once daily. Of the 66 patients who received budesonide alone, 25 (38%) achieved remission at 8 weeks. Although this proportion is

Study	Number of patients (budesonide arm)	Budesonide dose	Remission rate (% at 8 weeks)	
			Budesonide	Comparator
Greenberg et al., 1994 [8]	61	4.5 mg bid	51	20 (placebo)
Rutgeerts et al., 1994 [3]	88	9 mg OD	52	65 (prednisolone)
Campieri et al., 1997 [5]	58 OD/61 bid	9 mg OD/4.5 mg bid	60 OD/42 bid	60 (prednisolone)
Thomsen et al., 1998 [9]	93	9 mg OD	69	45 (mesalamine)
Steinhart et al., 2002 [10]	66	9 mg OD	38	N/A
Tremaine et al., 2002 [11]	80 OD/79 bid	9 mg OD/4.5 mg bid	48 OD/53 bid	33 (placebo)

Table 1. Controlled trials of budesonide (Entocort controlled ileal release) in active ileal and ileocecal Crohn's disease. bid: twice daily; N/A: not applicable; OD: once daily.

significantly lower than that observed in previous trials, the 95% confidence interval surrounding the point estimate includes the range of remission rates observed in previous studies. This raises the possibility that the observed remission rate might have been expected, given the normal variation observed in previous studies, and does not necessarily prove that the remission rates are as low as 38%.

Although these results do not negate the validity of previous trials, they do require refinement of the estimate of the true effectiveness of budesonide in ileal or ileocecal CD. Based upon available data, it is likely that remission can be expected in approximately half of "properly" selected patients with mild to moderate symptoms of ileal or ileocecal CD treated with budesonide, given as the Entocort CIR preparation.

Management of steroid dependency

Steroid dependency deters many physicians from initiating glucocorticoid therapy. The incidence of steroid dependency following a first course of therapy has been reported to be 36% by the end of 1 year [12].

Cortot et al. reported a trial in which they substituted budesonide for systemic glucocorticoid therapy in steroid-dependent patients with inactive CD [13]. In this study, patients with inactive CD – defined by a CD activity index (CDAI) of <200 – were randomized to receive placebo or budesonide 6 mg daily. Following initiation of the study treatment, prednisolone was tapered over a period of 4–10 weeks. Once completely tapered, the study medication (placebo or budesonide) was continued for another 12 weeks. After 13 weeks of prednisolone discontinuation, the proportion of patients experiencing a relapse – defined by an increase in CDAI score of >60 points – was twice as great in the placebo-treated patients compared with those receiving budesonide (65% vs. 32%, $P < 0.001$). In addition, glucocorticoid-associated side effects were reduced by approximately 50% following treatment conversion from prednisolone to budesonide.

Unfortunately, this study did not examine the efficacy or safety of long-term budesonide use as a means of sparing conventional glucocorticoids and maintaining remission. Although the ability to taper patients completely off conventional glucocorticoids is significant, the study period of 13 weeks was too short to have an important clinical impact on the long-term management of CD.

Maintenance of remission
Budesonide, 3 mg/day or 6 mg/day, does not prevent relapse over a 1-year period when used following induction of remission [6,14]. Green et al. have attempted to determine whether flexible dosing of budesonide, according to the patient's clinical status, might be a more effective way of maintaining remission compared with a fixed dose of 6 mg/day [15].

This study randomized patients to receive fixed budesonide dosing (6 mg/day) or flexible dosing, (3, 6, or 9 mg/day) according to their symptoms and their response to therapy. The investigators found no difference between the two arms with respect to the incidence of treatment failure (15% in the flexible-dosing group vs. 19% in the fixed-dose group) or the mean dose of budesonide received over the course of the study.

If the flexible-dosing strategy is indeed effective, it may not have been possible to determine it in this particular patient population due to the relatively low rate of relapse and treatment failure compared with previous studies of maintenance budesonide. Since the mean dose received was virtually identical in the two arms, it is not surprising that the clinical outcomes were similar.

Given the available data from earlier trials, it appears that budesonide is not effective at maintaining remission following induction of remission with an acute course of therapy. However, the study by Cortot et al. raises the possibility that budesonide may be a reasonable treatment strategy for patients who are dependent upon conventional glucocorticoids. Future studies should compare budesonide with alternative strategies, such as the use of immunomodulatory drugs, azathioprine, or 6-mercaptopurine, which have shown efficacy as long-term therapies in this patient population [16–18].

Pharmacogenomics

An area of great potential for the management of IBD is pharmacogenomics – the use of individual patient genetic profiles to predict the likelihood of response to a particular intervention. Investigators have examined the ability of various human leukocyte antigen (HLA)-DRB genotypes and interleukin-1 receptor antagonist genetic polymorphisms to predict the response to budesonide, in the context of a large randomized controlled trial [19]. The investigators found that the presence of a relatively rare HLA-DRB genotype – HLA-DR8 – was associated with nonresponse to budesonide. The presence of the HLA-DR8 allele was not associated with several disease features that were examined, eg, the presence of fistula or perianal disease, the need for surgery, or the disease site.

Although this study was only exploratory and hypothesis-generating, it supports the possibility of using patient genotypes to predict response to therapy, thereby maximizing the efficiency of treatment with glucocorticoids and other therapeutic agents.

Antibiotics

The use of antibiotics in primary and adjunctive therapy for CD and UC continues to be studied. This is primarily because the efficacy and safety of antibiotics in these settings is not well proven. Even in CD, where antibiotics are more widely considered to be effective, there continues to be controversy regarding their role in the overall therapeutic strategy, as discussed below.

Crohn's disease
Treatment of active disease
Studies have suggested that the nitroimidazole antibiotic metronidazole can be effective in the treatment of CD, particularly

when there is large-bowel involvement [20,21]. However, a trial by Sutherland et al. found no difference in the proportion of patients in remission among the groups treated with placebo or metronidazole, 10 or 20 mg/kg/day [21]. Critics of antibiotics have used these data to suggest that metronidazole, and antibiotics in general, have never demonstrated greater efficacy than placebo in the symptomatic treatment of active CD. Nonetheless, there is some degree of consistency among the studies; patients with large intestinal involvement seem to fare better with antibiotic treatment than those with small intestinal involvement only.

Sutherland et al. found a clear trend linking patient outcome to disease site, with the greatest improvement in mean CDAI relative to placebo in patients with large intestinal involvement only (206 points, $P = 0.05$), and the smallest improvement in those with small intestinal involvement only (40 points, $P =$ nonsignificant [21]). Those with combined small and large intestinal involvement showed intermediate improvement relative to placebo (103 points, $P = 0.05$). A similar trend was found in a study by Steinhart et al. that compared the use of budesonide alone with budesonide plus antibiotics (ciprofloxacin 500 mg/day and metronidazole 500 mg/day) in patients with active CD of the ileum, with or without involvement of the ascending colon [10]. The addition of antibiotics to budesonide therapy had no effect on the induction of remission in the total group of 134 patients. However, in the subset of patients with colonic disease, the addition of antibiotics produced a trend towards better outcomes at 8 weeks of therapy. Out of 33 patients with colonic disease, 9/17 (53%) of those receiving antibiotics achieved remission, whilst 4/16 (25%) of those receiving placebo had similarly positive outcomes ($P = 0.10$) (see **Figure 1**).

This study was not powered to detect a difference in response according to disease site, but the analysis of this prespecified subgroup agrees with trends observed in previous studies, and lends further weight to the contention that antibiotics are indeed effective in the treatment of colonic CD.

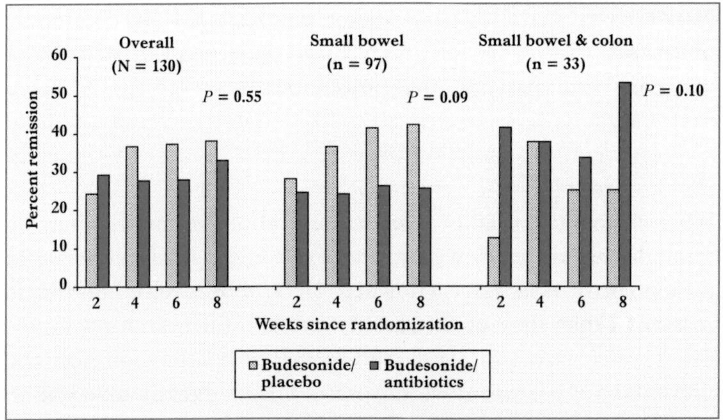

Figure 1. Proportion of patients in remission (Crohn's disease activity index <150) following randomization to receive budesonide (Entocort controlled ileal release capsules) plus placebo, or budesonide plus ciprofloxacin and metronidazole. Data are presented according to the site of disease. Reproduced with permission from WB Saunders Co. (*Gastroenterology* 2002;123:33–40).

Arnold et al. carried out a small, randomized, placebo-controlled trial of ciprofloxacin as adjuvant therapy in patients with treatment-resistant CD [22]. Patients with active CD (N = 47) were randomly assigned to receive placebo or ciprofloxacin for up to 6 months. Although the mean CDAI score was significantly lower in patients treated with ciprofloxacin (112 vs. 205, $P < 0.001$), the study was hampered by a much higher dropout rate in the placebo-treated patients (7/19, 37%) compared with that observed in the ciprofloxacin-treated patients (3/28, 11%). In addition, the placebo group had a mean baseline CDAI score that was 43 points higher than that of the ciprofloxacin-treated group (230 vs. 187). The trial was too small to comment on the efficacy of ciprofloxacin in the subgroup of patients with colonic CD, but it did provide some evidence that ciprofloxacin has a beneficial effect on CDAI scores.

There are no randomized, placebo-controlled studies of antibiotics in the therapy of perineal or fistulizing CD.

Nonetheless, metronidazole and/or ciprofloxacin are commonly prescribed in this scenario based upon anecdotal experience of clinicians and patients that antibiotics may reduce drainage from fistulae.

Relapse prevention

When medications fail or when complications occur, CD may be treated surgically. However, there is a considerable risk of postoperative relapse, even when all visibly involved bowel is resected at the time of surgery. As a result, the search continues for a safe, effective, and well-tolerated medication for the prevention of postoperative relapse of CD. Although mesalamine compounds appear to reduce the risk of postoperative relapse, the observed absolute risk reduction associated with their use is not high, and may not be considered clinically significant by many physicians and patients [23]. In a meta-analysis by Camma et al., the overall risk reduction was approximately 13% [23].

Most of the published experience with antibiotics revolves around the use of metronidazole [24]. However, metronidazole, particularly at the high doses (>10 mg/kg/day) used in some postoperative prophylactic studies, is associated with significant side effects and drug intolerance. Metallic taste, nausea, and vomiting are the most frequent dose-limiting side effects of the drug.

Ornidazole is a nitroimidazole antibiotic that is not currently available in North America. Rutgeerts et al. reported the results of a placebo-controlled, randomized trial of ornidazole (1 g/day) for the prevention of postoperative recurrence of CD in 80 patients following curative ileal or ileocolonic resection, and ileocolic anastomosis [25]. They found that ornidazole significantly reduced the occurrence of clinical relapse as defined by the presence of symptoms thought, by the physician, to be due to active CD (see **Table 2**). At 1 year, clinical relapse was observed in 8% of ornidazole-treated patients compared with 37% of placebo-treated patients ($P = 0.002$).

	Endoscopic recurrence (%)		Clinical recurrence (%)		
	3 months	12 months	12 months	24 months	36 months
Ornidazole 1 g/day	34	54	8	27	35
Placebo	59	79	37	45	48
P value	0.046	0.036	0.002	0.10	0.27

Table 2. Effect of ornidazole on endoscopic and clinical recurrence of Crohn's disease following surgery [25]. Reproduced with permission from WB Sauders Co. (*Gastroenterology* 2002;123:33–40).

Despite cessation of the study drug treatment after 1 year, there appeared to be a residual clinical benefit at 2 years. By this time, 27% of ornidazole-treated patients and 45% of placebo-treated patients had relapsed. Although this difference was not statistically significant, it is in keeping with the residual effect observed in a previous study of metronidazole [24]. Furthermore, a reduction in severe endoscopic recurrence was seen in the ornidazole-treated patients, and it was found that the occurrence of severe lesions was closely associated with clinical relapse. However, the use of ornidazole was not without side effects and intolerance. A greater proportion of ornidazole-treated patients withdrew from the study because of adverse reactions and intolerance compared with the placebo-treated patients. The adverse event profile of ornidazole is similar to that of metronidazole, with gastrointestinal intolerance predominating.

Antimycobacterial therapy
Some of the interest surrounding antibiotic therapy for CD stems from the suggestion that an atypical mycobacterial infection may somehow be involved in the etiology of CD [26,27]. Various investigators have tested several different antimycobacterial drug regimens, without any consistent effect observed between studies [28,29]. Leiper et al. reported an open series of 25 patients with

active CD who were treated for 12 weeks or more with clarithromycin, an antibiotic with activity against Mycobacteria [30]. The investigators reported a reduction in the median Harvey–Bradshaw index score from 9 (prior to therapy) to 5 (after 12 weeks of therapy). A Harvey–Bradshaw score ≤3 is generally felt to be equivalent to a CDAI score <150 (ie, remission). The median serum C-reactive protein level fell from 21.5 mg/L to 14.5 mg/L. Since there was no control arm in the study, it is difficult to determine whether the observed changes in clinical and laboratory parameters were due to intervention or to the natural fluctuation in disease activity. The reduction in Harvey–Bradshaw index score could also have been influenced by subject or observer bias.

Antimycobacterial therapy has also been tested in the prophylactic setting in order to prevent disease recurrence in patients with relatively quiescent disease. Goodgame et al. selected 31 patients at presumed high risk of relapse based upon the finding of increased intestinal permeability, measured by the lactulose–mannitol permeability test [31]. The patients were randomized to receive clarithromycin, 500 mg twice daily, and ethambutol, 15 mg/kg/day, or placebo, for 3 months, in addition to their usual therapy [31]. Over a period of 12 months, the investigators found no difference in intestinal permeability or disease activity between the two groups. It could be argued that the chosen drug regimen was inadequate, if the intent was to effectively eradicate an atypical Mycobacterium species Unfortunately, microbiologic outcomes were not examined in the trial.

Ulcerative colitis

Despite the fact that previous studies have provided inconsistent results, there has been ongoing interest in the use of antibiotics as adjunctive therapy for patients with moderate to severe UC [32–35]. More recently, Mantzaris et al. examined the use of intravenous (IV) ciprofloxacin as adjuvant therapy for patients with acute severe UC [36]. They randomly assigned 55 patients – admitted to hospital and treated with IV and rectal glucocorticoids – to receive IV ciprofloxacin, 400 mg twice daily, or placebo.

Significant improvement was observed in 79% and 77% of patients, respectively, suggesting that IV ciprofloxacin has no increased benefit beyond that observed with steroids alone.

These results are consistent with those observed in a previous study by the same group, in which patients with active UC were treated with oral ciprofloxacin or placebo in addition to their usual medical therapy [37]. Based upon the available evidence, the use of adjuvant antibiotic therapy cannot be recommended in UC.

Pouchitis

The use of antibiotics is relatively well accepted in the management of patients with acute pouchitis following colectomy and creation of an ileal pouch–anal anastomosis. Mimura et al. treated 44 patients with refractory or recurrent pouchitis with a combination of ciprofloxacin, 500 mg twice daily, and metronidazole, either 400 or 500 mg twice daily, for 4 weeks [38]. They observed clinical remission in 82% of their patients, determined by a pouchitis disease activity index total score ≤4. Although the study had no control group, it does support the commonly held impression that broad-spectrum antibiotics are effective in diminishing the symptoms of pouchitis.

5-aminosalicylic acid and derivatives

Crohn's disease

Interest continues in the development of effective, safe, and well-tolerated maintenance therapy for CD. It has long been hoped that 5-aminosalicylic acid/mesalamine would be such a therapeutic agent. A meta-analysis by Camma et al. has shown that mesalamine results in a 13% reduction in the risk of relapse in patients with CD following surgical resection [23].

More recently, the European Cooperative Crohn's Disease Study VI group examined the use of mesalamine (Pentasa), 4 g/day, in patients who had undergone surgical resection for CD [39]. A total of 318 patients were randomly assigned to receive mesalamine or placebo for 18 months. The investigators found recurrence rates of 31.4% and 24.5% in the placebo and mesalamine groups, respectively. This reduction in risk of recurrence (6.9%) was not statistically significant, and could not be considered clinically significant. However, in a *post hoc* analysis, the investigators found a statistically significant reduction in the risk of relapse in patients with isolated small intestinal disease (39.7% vs. 21.8%, $P = 0.02$).

Although the validity of a conclusion based upon *post hoc* analysis is rather suspect, the direction and magnitude of the risk reduction in patients with small intestinal disease is similar to that observed by McLeod et al. in a study of mesalamine 3 g/day for postoperative prophylaxis [40]. These results suggest that, in spite of the meta-analysis by Camma et al., postoperative mesalamine is a safe choice for prophylaxis against recurrent disease in patients with small intestinal CD.

The use of mesalamine for postoperative prophylaxis of CD, and for the prevention of relapse following medically-induced CD remissions, is very controversial. In their meta-analysis, Camma et al. showed a nonsignificant reduction in the risk of relapse (4.1%) when mesalamine was compared with placebo [23]. It has been argued that not all mesalamine controlled-release preparations are equivalent, and that evidence against the effectiveness of one preparation does not necessarily prove lack of effectiveness for another.

Olsalazine consists of two mesalamine molecules that are joined by a diazo bond and released by the action of bacterial azoreductase, primarily in the large intestine. It differs from most other mesalamine-containing preparations in that the mesalamine is not contained within a coating that results in time- or pH-dependent release of the drug.

Mahmud et al. studied the prophylactic effect of olsalazine, 2 g/day, in 328 patients with quiescent CD of the colon, or of the ileum and the colon [41]. In this study, the likelihood of experiencing a relapse over a 1-year period was equal in the patients randomized to receive olsalazine and those treated with placebo. In addition, the olsalazine-treated patients were more likely to experience gastrointestinal side effects and terminate treatment prematurely. Because of its primarily colonic release characteristic, olsalazine was not expected to provide an important benefit in patients with small intestinal CD. Nevertheless, the negative findings in this study provide further evidence against the use of mesalamine therapy for the prevention of CD relapse.

Ulcerative colitis

Treatment of active disease

The use of mesalamine to treat mild to moderate flares of disease activity, and to prevent relapse in patients with UC, has long been accepted as the cornerstone of therapy. In recent years, most clinical investigation surrounding the use of mesalamine has involved minor refinements of treatment strategies, and the introduction and testing of new carrier methods for delivering mesalamine to the inflamed colon.

Mansfield et al. randomized 50 patients with mild to moderately active UC to receive sulfasalazine, 3 g/day, or balsalazide, 6.75 g/day for 8 weeks [42]. Balsalazide consists of an inert carrier molecule bound to mesalamine by a diazo bond, which, in turn, is cleaved by colonic bacterial azoreductase. Balsalazide was better tolerated than sulfasalazine (nine patients receiving sulfasalazine and one patient receiving balsalazide dropped out due to side effects), and resulted in a greater likelihood of clinical remission.

These results were confirmed by another relatively small, randomized controlled trial of 57 patients with active UC [43]. In this study, patients with disease at all levels of severity were randomized to receive sulfasalazine, 3 g/day, or balsalazide, 6.75 g/day, and were followed for 12 weeks. A steady dose of topical or oral glucocorticoids was permitted throughout the study. The investigators found balsalazide to be associated with a lower rate of side effects than sulfasalazine. In the balsalazide arm, only 2/28 patients withdrew due to side effects, compared with 9/29 in the sulfasalazine arm.

It is likely that both of these studies were designed to highlight the safety and tolerability profile of balsalazide by comparing its use to that of sulfasalazine – a drug that is known for its potential side effects and gastrointestinal intolerance. Sulfasalazine therapy for mild to moderately active UC is no longer considered to be the standard first-line therapy in many centers and, therefore, comparison with a drug that is more commonly used (eg, mesalamine), would be more appropriate.

Such a comparison has been conducted. Levine et al. examined the use of balsalazide, 2.25 g/day or 6.75 g/day, with mesalamine, 2.4 g/day, in the treatment of a group of patients with mild to moderately active UC [44]. The 6.75 g dose of balsalazide is equivalent to 2.36 g of mesalamine. Despite the fact that the higher dose of balsalazide appeared to be more effective than the lower dose (73.7% improvement in Physician's Global Assessment compared with 51.3%, $P < 0.03$), it did not result in a better ultimate outcome than mesalamine.

The rectal administration of mesalamine in suppository or enema form has been recognized as first-line management of distal UC or proctitis [47]. However, some patients have difficulty holding the 60–100 mL enema volume, particularly when the rectum is very inflamed and, as a result, more irritable and less distensible.

It has been suggested that the use of combined oral and topical rectal mesalamine may improve response rates in patients with active UC [45]. A study of 130 patients with mild to moderately active UC found no difference in response between patients randomly assigned to receive oral mesalamine, 4 g/day, and those who received combined oral (2 g/day) and rectal (2 g/day) mesalamine in enema formats [46]. The earlier positive study [45] differed from this study in that the patients who received mesalamine therapy received a higher total dose of mesalamine than patients who received either oral or topical rectal mesalamine alone. These results do not support the routine use of combined therapy, except perhaps for those patients with prominent symptoms of rectal inflammation.

The rectal administration of mesalamine in the formulation of a foam could potentially improve retention and mucosal contact time. Pokrotnieks et al. studied the use of a mesalamine foam enema preparation in a randomized, placebo-controlled trial in 111 patients with mild to moderately active ulcerative proctitis, proctosigmoiditis, or left-sided colitis [48]. The enemas contained 2 g mesalamine and were administered daily for 6 weeks. Clinical and endoscopic remissions were observed in 65% and 57%, respectively, of patients treated with mesalamine foam enemas. This compared favorably with clinical and endoscopic remission rates of 40% and 37% in the placebo enema-treated patients ($P < 0.01$ for clinical remission, $P = 0.047$ for endoscopic remission).

More recently, Malchow and Gertz studied another mesalamine foam enema preparation (Claversal, 2 g/day), and compared it with a standard 4 g mesalamine liquid enema in patients with distal UC [49]. A total of 264 patients, with disease extent anywhere between the splenic flexure and 12 cm from the anus, were randomized to one of two treatment arms for 4 weeks. In the per protocol analysis, 64.9% of patients in the foam enema group and 69.5% of patients in the liquid enema group achieved clinical remission. No statistically significant difference was found when the groups were analyzed on an intent-to-treat basis. Interestingly, the reporting of adverse events considered to have been possibly or probably associated with the study medication was more frequent in the foam group (14/133 vs. 4/131). Based upon these results, the precise role of mesalamine foam enemas in the treatment of left-sided UC remains to be determined.

Maintenance of remission
It is well recognized that sulfasalazine and mesalamine are effective in maintaining remission in patients with UC. Despite

claims that the various mesalamine compounds differ in their efficacy, or differ when measured against sulfasalazine, there is no controlled evidence to support these claims [50].

Newer mesalamine delivery methods, eg, balsalazide, have been tested against controlled-release forms of mesalamine for their ability to maintain remission. In a study of 133 patients, Kruis et al. found that balsalazide, 1.5 g twice daily, was as effective as mesalamine, 0.5 g three times daily, in maintaining disease remission over a 26-week study period [51]. Balsalazide, 3 g twice daily, was found to be superior to both low-dose balsalazide and mesalamine with remission rates of 77.5%, 43.8%, and 56.8%, respectively ($P = 0.006$). This supports the hypothesis that a dose effect for mesalamine exists with respect to the maintenance of remission, and that using higher doses of the mesalamine product might achieve significantly higher remission rates.

Cyclosporine

Pharmacotherapy

A small, placebo-controlled trial demonstrated that IV cyclosporine produced symptomatic improvement in patients with acute severe UC who were admitted to hospital and were not responding to IV glucocorticoid therapy [52]. It was also shown that these cyclosporine-treated patients were able to avoid colectomy. However, the routine use of cyclosporine has not been widely adopted in many centers because of concerns regarding toxicity and the relatively high rate of colectomy observed with long-term follow-up [53,54]. It has been argued that some of the toxicity associated with the use of IV cyclosporine in the acute setting, particularly the occurrence of opportunistic infections, is attributable to the concomitant or preceding use of high-dose glucocorticoids.

D'Haens et al. carried out a study comparing IV cyclosporine monotherapy, 4 mg/kg/day, with IV methylprednisolone, 40 mg/day, in 30 patients with acute severe colitis [55]. Response was observed in 64% and 53% of patients, respectively, with no major drug toxicity seen in either group. Furthermore, 78% of patients who initially responded to cyclosporine maintained remission at 1 year, compared with only 37% of patients treated with steroids.

Although this study suggests that the use of cyclosporine monotherapy may be relatively safe, and appears to provide good medium-term prognosis, the sample size was too small to draw firm conclusions. Additional larger studies with long-term follow-up are required to define the role of cyclosporine in the management of acute severe UC.

Azathioprine

Pharmacotherapy

The use of purine analogs in the long-term management of CD is gaining increasing acceptance among physicians, and is supported by evidence from controlled clinical trials [18]. Determining the appropriate duration of therapy and the timing of drug discontinuation is a common issue that arises with the use of these medications.

Lemann et al. have examined this issue in the context of a controlled clinical trial in which patients who were stable on azathioprine for at least 42 months, without a disease flare, were randomized to receive either continued azathioprine or placebo for another 18 months [56]. Relapse occurred in nine of the 43 placebo-treated patients and three of the 40 azathioprine-treated patients. Although the observed difference in recurrence rates was significant, the rate observed in the placebo group was still relatively low and, given this information, some patients might opt to discontinue therapy.

The investigators also found that an elevated serum C-reactive protein level was predictive of relapse. In patients who have been clinically stable on long-term azathioprine, and who have normal serum C-reactive protein levels, drug discontinuation may be a reasonable option.

Conclusion

The introduction of newer unconventional or biological therapies for the treatment of IBD is likely to provide advances in the management of patients. However, decisions regarding the appropriate situations in which to use these newer agents will be dependent upon full knowledge of the uses and limitations of existing conventional therapies such as 5-aminosalicylic acid, glucocorticoids, antibiotics, and immunomodulators. It is unlikely that newer therapies will completely supplant conventional therapies in the near future. It is more likely that the way in which these therapies are used will be modified over time.

References

1. Modigliani R, Mary JY, Simon JF et al. Clinical, biological, and endoscopic picture of attacks of Crohn's disease. Evolution on prednisolone. Groupe d'Etude Therapeutique des Affections Inflammatoires Digestives. *Gastroenterology* 1990;98:811–8.
2. Singleton JW, Law DH, Kelley ML Jr et al. National Cooperative Crohn's Disease Study: adverse reactions to study drugs. *Gastroenterology* 1979;77:870–82.
3. Rutgeerts P, Lofberg R, Malchow H et al. A comparison of budesonide with prednisolone for active Crohn's disease. *N Engl J Med* 1994;331:842–5.
4. Lofberg R, Danielsson A, Suhr O et al. Oral budesonide versus prednisolone in patients with active extensive and left-sided ulcerative colitis. *Gastroenterology* 1996;110:1713–8.
5. Campieri M, Ferguson A, Doe W et al. Oral budesonide is as effective as oral prednisolone in active Crohn's disease. The Global Budesonide Study Group. *Gut* 1997;41:209–14.
6. Ferguson A, Campieri M, Doe W et al. Oral budesonide as maintenance therapy in Crohn's disease – results of a 12-month study. Global Budesonide Study Group. *Aliment Pharmacol Ther* 1998;12:175–83.
7. Lundin P, Naber T, Nilsson M et al. Effect of food on the pharmacokinetics of budesonide controlled ileal release capsules in patients with active Crohn's disease. *Aliment Pharmacol Ther* 2001;15:45–51.
8. Greenberg GR, Feagan BG, Martin F et al. Oral budesonide for active Crohn's disease. Canadian Inflammatory Bowel Disease Study Group. *N Engl J Med* 1994;331:836–41.
9. Thomsen OO, Cortot A, Jewell D et al. A comparison of budesonide and mesalamine for active Crohn's disease. International Budesonide-Mesalamine Study Group. *N Engl J Med* 1998;339:370–4.
10. Steinhart AH, Feagan BG, Wong CJ et al. Combined budesonide and antibiotic therapy for active Crohn's disease: a randomized controlled trial. *Gastroenterology* 2002;123:33–40.

11. Tremaine WJ, Hanauer SB, Katz S et al. Budesonide CIR capsules (once or twice daily divided-dose) in active Crohn's disease: a randomized placebo-controlled study in the United States. *Am J Gastroenterol* 2002;97:1748–54.

12. Munkholm P, Langholz E, Davidsen M et al. Frequency of glucocorticoid resistance and dependency in Crohn's disease. *Gut* 1994;35:360–2.

13. Cortot A, Colombel JF, Rutgeerts P et al. Switch from systemic steroids to budesonide in steroid dependent patients with inactive Crohn's disease. *Gut* 2001;48:186–90.

14. Greenberg GR, Feagan BG, Martin F et al. Oral budesonide as maintenance treatment for Crohn's disease: a placebo-controlled, dose-ranging study. Canadian Inflammatory Bowel Disease Study Group. *Gastroenterology* 1996;110:45–51.

15. Green JR, Lobo AJ, Giaffer M et al. Maintenance of Crohn's disease over 12 months: fixed versus flexible dosing regimen using budesonide controlled ileal release capsules. *Aliment Pharmacol Ther* 2001;15:1331–41.

16. Candy S, Wright J, Gerber M et al. A controlled double blind study of azathioprine in the management of Crohn's disease. *Gut* 1995;37:674–8.

17. Lemann M, Bonhomme P, Bitoun A et al. Treatment of Crohn's disease with azathioprine or 6-mercaptopurine. Retrospective study of 126 cases. *Gastroenterol Clin Biol* 1990;14:548–54.

18. Pearson DC, May GR, Fick GH et al. Azathioprine and 6-mercaptopurine in Crohn's disease. A meta-analysis. *Ann Intern Med* 1995;123:132–42.

19. Gelbmann CM, Rogler G, Gierend M et al. Association of HLA-DR genotypes and IL-1ra gene polymorphism with treatment failure of budesonide and disease patterns in Crohn's disease. *Eur J Gastroenterol Hepatol* 2001;13:1431–7.

20. Ursing B, Alm T, Barany F et al. A comparative study of metronidazole and sulfasalazine for active Crohn's disease: the cooperative Crohn's disease study in Sweden. II. Result. *Gastroenterology* 1982;83:550–62.

21. Sutherland L, Singleton J, Sessions J et al. Double blind, placebo controlled trial of metronidazole in Crohn's disease. *Gut* 1991;32:1071–5.

22. Arnold GL, Beaves MR, Pryjdun VO et al. Preliminary study of ciprofloxacin in active Crohn's disease. *Inflamm Bowel Dis* 2002;8:10–15.

23. Camma C, Giunta M, Rosselli M et al. Mesalamine in the maintenance treatment of Crohn's disease: a meta-analysis adjusted for confounding variables. *Gastroenterology* 1997;113:1465–73.

24. Rutgeerts P, Hiele M, Geboes K et al. Controlled trial of metronidazole treatment for prevention of Crohn's recurrence after ileal resection. *Gastroenterology* 1995;108:1617–21.

25. Rutgeerts P, Van Assche G, D'Haens G et al. Ornidazol for prophylaxis of postoperative Crohn's disease: final results of a double blind placebo controlled trial. *Gastroenterology* 2002;122:80A.

26. El-Zaatari FA, Naser SA, Hulten K et al. Characterization of Mycobacterium paratuberculosis p36 antigen and its seroreactivities in Crohn's disease. *Curr Microbiol* 1999;39:115–9.

27. Lisby G, Andersen J, Engbaek K et al. Mycobacterium paratuberculosis in intestinal tissue from patients with Crohn's disease demonstrated by a nested primer polymerase chain reaction. *Scand J Gastroenterol* 1994;29:923–9.

28. Hulten K, Almashhrawi A, El-Zaatari FA et al. Antibacterial therapy for Crohn's disease: a review emphasizing therapy directed against mycobacteria. *Dig Dis Sci* 2000;45:445–56.

29. Prantera C, Kohn A, Mangiarotti R et al. Antimycobacterial therapy in Crohn's disease: results of a controlled, double-blind trial with a multiple antibiotic regimen. *Am J Gastroenterol* 1994;89:513–8.

30. Leiper K, Morris AI, Rhodes JM. Open label trial of oral clarithromycin in active Crohn's disease. *Aliment Pharmacol Ther* 2000;14:801–6.

31. Goodgame RW, Kimball K, Akram S et al. Randomized controlled trial of clarithromycin and ethambutol in the treatment of Crohn's disease. *Aliment Pharmacol Ther* 2001;15:1861–6.

32. Burke DA, Axon AT, Clayden SA et al. The efficacy of tobramycin in the treatment of ulcerative colitis. *Aliment Pharmacol Ther* 1990;4:123–9.

33. Lobo AJ, Burke DA, Sobala GM et al. Oral tobramycin in ulcerative colitis: effect on maintenance of remission. *Aliment Pharmacol Ther* 1993;7:155–8.

34. Mantzaris GJ, Hatzis A, Kontogiannis P et al. Intravenous tobramycin and metronidazole as an adjunct to corticosteroids in acute, severe ulcerative colitis. *Am J Gastroenterol* 1994;89:43–6.

35. Turunen UM, Farkkila MA, Hakala K et al. Long-term treatment of ulcerative colitis with ciprofloxacin: a prospective, double-blind, placebo-controlled study. *Gastroenterology* 1998;115:1072–8.

36. Mantzaris GJ, Petraki K, Archavlis E et al. A prospective randomized controlled trial of intravenous ciprofloxacin as an adjunct to corticosteroids in acute, severe ulcerative colitis. *Scand J Gastroenterol* 2001;36:971–4.

37. Mantzaris GJ, Archavlis E, Christoforidis P et al. A prospective randomized controlled trial of oral ciprofloxacin in acute ulcerative colitis. *Am J Gastroenterol* 1997;92:454–6.

38. Mimura T, Rizzello F, Helwig U et al. Four-week open-label trial of metronidazole and ciprofloxacin for the treatment of recurrent or refractory pouchitis. *Aliment Pharmacol Ther* 2002;16:909–17.

39. Lochs H, Mayer M, Fleig WE et al. Prophylaxis of postoperative relapse in Crohn's disease with mesalamine: European Cooperative Crohn's Disease Study VI. *Gastroenterology* 2000;118:264–73.

40. McLeod RS, Wolff BG, Steinhart AH et al. Prophylactic mesalamine treatment decreases postoperative recurrence of Crohn's disease. *Gastroenterology* 1995;109:404–13.

41. Mahmud N, Kamm MA, Dupas JL et al. Olsalazine is not superior to placebo in maintaining remission of inactive Crohn's colitis and ileocolitis: a double blind, parallel, randomised, multicentre study. *Gut* 2001;49:552–6.

42. Mansfield JC, Giaffer MH, Cann PA et al. A double-blind comparison of balsalazide, 6.75 g, and sulfasalazine, 3 g, as sole therapy in the management of ulcerative colitis. *Aliment Pharmacol Ther* 2002;16:69–77.

43. Green JR, Mansfield JC, Gibson JA et al. A double-blind comparison of balsalazide, 6.75 g daily, and sulfasalazine, 3 g daily, in patients with newly diagnosed or relapsed active ulcerative colitis. *Aliment Pharmacol Ther* 2002;16:61–8.

44. Levine DS, Riff DS, Pruitt R et al. A randomized, double blind, dose-response comparison of balsalazide (6.75 g), balsalazide (2.25 g), and mesalamine (2.4 g) in the treatment of active, mild-to-moderate ulcerative colitis. *Am J Gastroenterol* 2002;97:1398–407.

45. Safdi M, DeMicco M, Sninsky C et al. A double-blind comparison of oral versus rectal mesalamine versus combination therapy in the treatment of distal ulcerative colitis. *Am J Gastroenterol* 1997;92:1867–71.

46. Vecchi M, Meucci G, Gionchetti P et al. Oral versus combination mesalazine therapy in active ulcerative colitis: a double-blind, double-dummy, randomized multicentre study. *Aliment Pharmacol Ther* 2001;15:251–6.

47. Marshall JK, Irvine EJ. Rectal corticosteroids versus alternative treatments in ulcerative colitis: a meta-analysis. *Gut* 1997;40:775–81.

48. Pokrotnieks J, Marlicz K, Paradowski L et al. Efficacy and tolerability of mesalazine foam enema (Salofalk foam) for distal ulcerative colitis: a double-blind, randomized, placebo-controlled study. *Aliment Pharmacol Ther* 2000;14:1191–8.

49. Malchow H, Gertz B. A new mesalazine foam enema (Claversal Foam) compared with a standard liquid enema in patients with active distal ulcerative colitis. *Aliment Pharmacol Ther* 2002;16:415–23.

50. Sutherland LR, May GR, Shaffer EA. Sulphasalazine revisited: a meta-analysis of 5-aminosalicylic acid in the treatment of ulcerative colitis. *Ann Intern Med* 1993; 118:540–9.

51. Kruis W, Schreiber S, Theuer D et al. Low dose balsalazide (1.5 g twice daily) and mesalazine (0.5 g three times daily) maintained remission of ulcerative colitis but high dose balsalazide (3.0 g twice daily) was superior in preventing relapses. *Gut* 2001;49: 783–9.

52. Lichtiger S, Present DH, Kornbluth A et al. Cyclosporine in severe ulcerative colitis refractory to steroid therapy. *N Engl J Med* 1994;330:1841–5.

53. Atkinson KA, McDonald JW, Lamba B et al. Intravenous cyclosporine for severe attacks of ulcerative colitis: a survey of Canadian gastroenterologists. *Can J Gastroenterol* 1997;11:583–7.

54. Cohen RD, Stein R, Hanauer SB. Intravenous cyclosporin in ulcerative colitis: a five-year experience. *Am J Gastroenterol* 1999;94:1587–92.

55. D'Haens G, Lemmens L, Geboes K et al. Intravenous cyclosporine versus intravenous corticosteroids as single therapy for severe attacks of ulcerative colitis. *Gastroenterology* 2001;120:1323–9.

56. Lemann M, Bouhnik Y, Colombel JF et al. Randomized double-blind placebo-controlled multicenter azathioprine withdrawal trial in Crohn's disease. *Gastroenterology* 2002;122:23A.

at weeks 0, 2, and 6. Of the patients who received 5 mg/kg and 10 mg/kg infliximab, 68% and 56%, respectively, achieved the primary endpoint (>50% reduction in the number of draining fistulae) compared with 26% of the patients in the placebo group ($P = 0.002; P = 0.02$). Closure of all fistulae was noted in 55% of patients who received 5 mg/kg of infliximab, 38% of patients who received 10 mg/kg infliximab, and 13% of patients who received placebo.

Preliminary data from the ACCENT II study – a multicenter, randomized trial to assess the efficacy of maintenance infliximab in fistulizing CD – are now available [8]. This study evaluated the efficacy of maintenance dosing (5 mg/kg at weeks 0, 2, 6, and then every 8 weeks) with infliximab in sustaining fistula closure, compared with a single, three-dose induction regimen (5 mg/kg at weeks 0, 2, and 6). All patients (N = 307) enrolled in the study had single or multiple draining fistulae of ≥3 months duration preceding screening.

Of the 282 patients who completed the study through to week 14, 69% had closure of at least 50% of draining fistulae after receiving a 5 mg/kg dose of infliximab at weeks 0, 2, and 6. Responders were then randomized to receive placebo or 5 mg/kg of infliximab every 8 weeks through to week 46. A full report of these results is anticipated shortly.

Infliximab in the treatment of UC
Much less is known about the role of infliximab in the treatment of UC, despite *in vitro* and animal (cotton-top tamarin) data that support a potential role for TNF-α in the pathogenesis of this disease. A study by Sands et al. reported 11 patients with severely active, steroid-refractory UC who were treated with infliximab (n = 8) or placebo (n = 3) in a double-blind fashion [19]. The study was terminated prematurely due to slow enrollment. However, 50% of patients who received infliximab (single infusion) achieved a clinical response at 2 weeks compared with 0% of the placebo-treated patients.

Adverse effect	Prevalence (%) [ref.]	Possible preventive measures
Infusion reactions	20–27 [7,25]	Pretreat with glucocorticoids
Serious infection	30 [7]	Vigilance for abscesses
Tuberculosis	0.057 [28]	Pretreatment with purified protein derivative skin test ± chest x-ray
Antichimeric antibodies	14–68 [7,23,25]	Use of concurrent immunosuppressants
Antinuclear antibodies	34–56 [7,26]	Not usually clinically significant
Antidouble-stranded DNA antibodies	9–34 [7,26,27]	Not usually clinically significant

Table 3. Unique adverse events with infliximab therapy.

Chey et al. evaluated single infusion infliximab (5 mg/kg) among eight patients with UC, who were refractory to conventional therapy [20]. All patients demonstrated clinical improvement at 1-week follow-up ($P < 0.01$). None of the patients relapsed, although they were all maintained on additional immuno-suppressive regimens, including 6-mercaptopurine. Additional open-label trials have also demonstrated the potential role of infliximab therapy for glucocorticoid sparing and short-term avoidance of colectomy.

Probert et al. evaluated a single infusion regimen of infliximab (5 mg/kg) compared with placebo in 42 patients with glucocorticoid-resistant UC. At 2, 6, and 8 weeks after infusion, infliximab proved to be no better than placebo at inducing a clinical remission (36% vs. 30%, respectively) [21].

Larger studies are required to clarify the role of infliximab in the management of UC. These preliminary data are not supportive of its current use.

Adverse effects

The central role of TNF-α in maintaining immunologic homeostasis has led to a relatively unique set of adverse effects associated with its inhibition (see **Table 3**). However, infliximab appears to be safe and well tolerated.

In the ACCENT I trial, the prevalence of serious adverse events was no different among patients in group 1 (29%) compared with those in groups 2 and 3 (28% and 22%, respectively). However, infusion reactions were significantly more prevalent among infliximab-treated patients compared with controls (21% vs. 9%, respectively). The incidence of intestinal stenosis was no different among the groups in this study: 3% in group 1, 2% in group 2, and 3% in group 3.

Human antichimeric antibody formation
As a chimeric monoclonal antibody, infliximab may induce the formation of neutralizing antibodies. In the ACCENT I trial, formation of human antichimeric antibodies (HACA) was shown to result in loss of response to infliximab, infusion reactions, and, in some patients, delayed hypersensitivity-type reactions, particularly after a "drug holiday" [22].

The prevalence of HACA is difficult to assess given the interference of biologically active infliximab with the currently used assay; indeterminate assays have been reported to be as high as 68% [23].

In ACCENT I, 14% of 442 patients evaluated for HACA were described as clearly positive, 40% were negative, and 46% were inconclusive [7]. The prevalence of HACA was highest among patients who were randomized to placebo after week 2 (28%), compared with only 6% among patients who received 10 mg/kg infliximab every 8 weeks for maintenance.

Patients on concomitant glucocorticoid and immunomodulatory therapy had the lowest prevalence of HACA (6%) compared with those who were not receiving these agents (18%). Furthermore, data from ACCENT I supported the observation that infusion reactions were more prevalent in HACA-positive patients (17% vs. 8%). A recent report concluded that premedication of infliximab infusions with hydrocortisone can reduce the prevalence of HACA at 16 weeks, with 31% of hydrocortisone-treated patients having measurable HACA compared with 50% of placebo-treated patients ($P = 0.03$) [24].

In a survey of 125 patients with CD who were treated with infliximab infusions (mean 3.9 infusions/patient), 61% of patients had detectable levels of HACA (lower limit of detection 1.40 μg/mL) [25]. Prior to infusion, concentrations of $\geq$8.0 μg/mL predicted a shorter duration of response compared with patients with concentrations of <8.0 μg/mL (35 days vs. 71 days, $P < 0.001$). Furthermore, individuals with the higher concentrations carried a higher risk of infusion reactions (relative risk of 2.40, $P < 0.001$). Patients who had infusion reactions had a shorter duration of response (median 38.5 days vs. 65 days, $P < 0.001$). As noted in other studies, concomitant immunosuppressive therapy was predictive of low titers of antibodies against infliximab ($P < 0.001$) and high concentrations of infliximab 4 weeks after an infusion ($P < 0.001$).

Other antibody formation
The development of other autoantibodies has been evaluated in infliximab-treated patients. The evidence suggests that the prevalence of antinuclear antibodies (ANA) and antidouble-stranded DNA (anti-dsDNA) antibodies amongst all patients treated with infliximab is 34% and 9%, respectively [26].

In ACCENT I, the frequency of ANA and anti-dsDNA antibodies was significantly higher in infliximab-treated patients (56% and 34%, respectively) compared with placebo-treated patients (35% and 11%, respectively) [7]. In this study, only two patients were felt to have developed clinical evidence of a lupus-like syndrome, which is consistent with other experiences [27].

Infection

Serious infection is the greatest concern in the short- and long-term follow-up of patients treated with infliximab. The role of TNF-α in mediating immune responses to intracellular pathogens, including *Mycobacterium* species, *Listeria monocytogenes*, and *Histoplasma capsulatum*, has been well described. Of the 175,000 patients treated with infliximab (mostly for CD and rheumatoid arthritis), there have been 101 cases of tuberculosis. This has made pretreatment testing with a purified protein derivative (PPD) skin test an essential component of the evaluation of patients before implementing infliximab therapy [7,28]. If the patient has an abnormal PPD, then a chest x-ray is also required.

In ACCENT I, infection requiring antimicrobial treatment was noted in 32% of all patients, with no difference among placebo-treated and infliximab-treated patients [7]. Serious infections occurred in 4% of all patients, and were noted equally among the three groups. One patient developed tuberculosis. Other series have shown slightly higher rates of overall infection among infliximab-treated compared with placebo-treated patients (32% vs. 22%) [26].

Neoplasia

The incidence of neoplasia has been evaluated in patients undergoing treatment with infliximab. In ACCENT I, a total of six cancers developed, including breast cancer, renal cell cancer, bladder cancer, an epithelial cell skin cancer, a basal cell skin cancer, and a natural killer cell lymphoma [7]. In this study, the lack of a pure placebo control group and long-term follow-up make it difficult to draw firm conclusions about the relationship between infliximab treatment and neoplasia. Long-term evaluation in a large cohort with an appropriate comparator population may provide a conclusive answer.

Infliximab and pregnancy

There have been 42 women who have become pregnant while being treated with infliximab. As yet, there have been no reports of excessive or unusual teratogenic events [29]. Despite this observation, infliximab cannot be recommended for routine use among pregnant patients with CD.

CDP571

Molecular mechanism

CDP571 was genetically engineered as a humanized form of anti-TNF-α antibody, with the theoretic advantage of being less immunogenic. The molecule was constructed by linking the complementary-determining region (CDR) of a murine antihuman TNF-α moiety with a human IgG$_4$ antibody.

As with infliximab, CDP571 is capable of neutralizing both soluble and transmembrane-bound TNF-α. However, complement and antibody-dependent cell-mediated cytotoxicity is less efficient with CDP571 due to the fragment crystallizable (Fc) component of the IgG$_4$ molecule. It is unclear whether infliximab and CDP571 are equally effective inducers of T-cell apoptosis.

Clinical trials

The experience with CDP571 in IBD therapy is limited to a few clinical trials. Stack et al. evaluated the efficacy of CDP571 in 31 patients with moderately active CD [30]. Patients were randomly assigned in a 2:1 design (treatment:placebo). The treatment arm received a single infusion of CDP571 at 5 mg/kg and was followed for 2 weeks. At follow-up, there was a significant reduction in CDAI from 262 (median) at baseline to 167 at 2 weeks. Six patients achieved clinical remission. There were also notable reductions in C-reactive protein and serum orosomucoid, which are classic serum biomarkers of inflammation.

Feagan et al. evaluated 71 glucocorticoid-dependent patients with moderate to severe CD [31]. Patients were randomized to receive sequential doses of CDP571, starting with a single infusion of 20 mg/kg and then 10 mg/kg every 8 weeks through to 16 weeks, or placebo. At week 16, 44% of CDP571-treated patients had

The largest study evaluating ISIS-2302 was reported by Yacyshyn et al [54]. This randomized, double-blind, placebo-controlled study evaluated ISIS-2302 in 299 patients with steroid-dependent CD. An IV regimen of ISIS-2302 (2 mg/kg) or placebo three times weekly for 2 or 4 weeks was given. At week 14, ISIS-2302-treated patients (2-week and 4-week regimens combined) were more frequently glucocorticoid-free than placebo-treated patients (78% vs. 64%, respectively, $P = 0.032$).

Targeted blockade of leukocyte trafficking remains a promising area of molecular development and clinical investigation in IBD. Further studies of dose and interval optimization are clearly warranted before these therapies enter into the therapeutic paradigm of IBD.

Th1 polarization

Numerous studies have demonstrated a consistent pattern of Th1-type cell predominance in the affected mucosa and submucosa of patients with CD. This is characterized by the preferential expression of IL-2, IL-12, IL-18, IFN-γ, TNF-α, and IL-1β by infiltrating lymphocytes and macrophages. At present, specific determinants of this immunologic phenotype remain unclear, though it appears that this condition is essential for maintaining disease activity.

Attempts to "rebalance" the state of Th cell activation within the mucosa and submucosa have resulted in the development of targeted therapeutic agents to reset this milieu. This is one of the primary mechanisms by which TNF-α inhibition appears to successfully treat CD.

Experimental evidence also suggests that thalidomide and sulfasalazine can inhibit macrophage-derived IL-12. Antibodies directed against IL-12, IFN-γ, IL-2 receptor, and IL-18 have all been shown to be effective in animal models of colitis [55,56]. There are currently no human data with anti-IL-12 or anti-IL-18 agents.

HuZAF

HuZAF is a humanized monoclonal antibody against IFN-γ. Rutgeerts et al. reported a placebo-controlled, double-blind, dose-escalation study with this agent in 28 patients with moderately active CD [57]. They found that a single IV dose of 4 mg/kg resulted in a 71% remission rate at 4 weeks follow-up. Adverse effects were evenly distributed across active- and placebo-treated patients. A larger randomized controlled trial is currently underway.

Interleukin-10

IL-10 has been shown to exert numerous anti-inflammatory actions, and has long been felt to be a potential target in CD. A study has shown that a low ileal IL-10 mRNA concentration is a strong predictor of endoscopic recurrence among patients with CD who have undergone surgical resection [58].

A dose-finding study was reported by van Deventer et al [59]. A total of 46 patients with steroid-resistant CD were treated with daily IV boluses of recombinant human (rh)IL-10 (0.5–25 μg/kg) or placebo for 7 days. At 3 weeks of follow-up, 50% of rhIL-10-treated patients were in remission compared with 23% of placebo-treated patients. Glucocorticoid sparing was not evident. Adverse effects appeared to be well distributed across the active- and placebo-treated arms.

Schreiber et al. performed a prospective, multicenter, randomized, double-blind, placebo-controlled investigation of rhIL-10 among 329 steroid-refractory CD patients [60]. Patients received SC rhIL-10 daily for 28 days, with doses ranging from 1 to 20 μg/kg, or placebo. At 4 weeks' follow-up, there was no statistically significant difference in remission rates between placebo and active-treatment arms, though there was a trend towards clinical improvement. They also noted that responders to rhIL-10 had evidence of nuclear factor (NF)-κB (an important transcriptional regulator of multiple proinflammatory cytokines) reduction as measured by Western blot analysis of ileal biopsy lysates. A notable finding in this study was evidence of dose-dependent (>8 μg/kg) anemia and thrombocytopenia.

Fedorak et al. conducted a 24-week trial of rhIL-10 in 95 patients with mild to moderate CD [61]. They used a similar dose-escalation scheme to Schreiber et al. The primary endpoint – remission at day 29 – was observed in 29.4% of patients who received rhIL-10 (5 μg/kg) compared with 0% of the placebo-treated patients (intention-to-treat analysis).

Higher doses were less effective, which supports experimental evidence suggesting that high concentrations of IL-10 may promote IFN-γ secretion. Asymptomatic and reversible reductions in hemoglobin and platelet counts were seen in 25% and 7% of active-treatment patients, respectively, compared with 18% and 0% among placebo-treated patients. Autoantibodies against IL-10 were not observed.

A larger study by Fedorak et al. involving 373 patients with steroid-dependent CD also failed to show significant differences in remission rates. In this study, patients were randomized to a 26-week course of rhIL-10 (4 μg/kg or 8 μg/kg) or placebo. At 28 weeks, intention-to-treat analysis demonstrated no significant difference in the prednisone withdrawal and clinical remission rates between the three treatment arms: 4 μg/kg (25%), 8 μg/kg (32%), and placebo (29%) [62].

The utility of rhIL-10 to prevent postoperative recurrence of CD after ileal or ileocolonic resection has also been investigated. Colombel et al. randomized 65 patients to receive SC rhIL-10 (4 μg/kg or 8 μg/kg) or placebo, starting 2 weeks after surgery [63]. Endoscopic recurrences were similar in each group at 12 weeks follow-up: 52% in the placebo arm and 46% in the rhIL-10 arm.

These results have led to alternative treatment strategies involving rhIL-10, using modified drug delivery systems. Ongoing studies are evaluating both topical and viral vector-delivered drugs, including genetically modified *Lactococcus* and adenoviral vectors [64,65].

Daclizumab and basiliximab

IL-2 is a key mediator in the differentiation of Th cells into Th1 cells. There are currently two monoclonal antibodies under evaluation, both of which target neutralization of IL-2 by blocking the binding of IL-2 to its receptor, IL-2R. Daclizumab is a humanized antibody (>90% human and 10% mouse Ig) and basiliximab is a chimeric antibody (70% human Ig and 30% mouse Ig).

Limited data with daclizumab show short-term efficacy in uncontrolled, open-label trials of small numbers of patients with UC [66]. In this trial, 10 patients with UC were treated with daclizumab, 1 mg/kg twice with a 4-week interval. At 8 weeks follow-up, improved median clinical and endoscopic scores were noted ($P < 0.005$ and $P < 0.01$, respectively). Quality of life, as assessed by the IBDQ, increased after therapy ($P < 0.05$). There are currently no data available for the use of basiliximab in IBD.

Growth factors

Epidermal growth factor (EGF) and keratinocyte growth factor (KGF) have been shown to stimulate cell proliferation in the gastrointestinal (GI) tract. KGF quantity and distribution appear to be abnormal in patients with IBD. KGF mRNA levels are increased in inflamed IBD tissue in comparison with control tissues. In normal tissue, KGF mRNA is localized to the mesenchymal cells at the tip of the villi in the small intestine and directly underlying the mature enterocytes in the colon. In IBD tissue, it is present throughout the lamina propria [67].

In the form of an enema, rhEGF was evaluated in an open-label, placebo-controlled trial in 23 patients with active left-sided UC [68]. At 4 weeks of follow-up, remission was noted in 82% of patients treated with rhEG compared with 25% of placebo-treated patients ($P < 0.001$). RhKGF-2, repifermin, was recently evaluated in a randomized, dose-escalating, double-blind, placebo-controlled trial involving 88 patients with active UC [69]. Treatment arms included: 1 µg/kg (n = 11), 5 µg/kg (n = 11), 10 µg/kg (n = 12), 25 µg/kg (n = 12), 50 µg/kg (n = 14), and placebo infusion (n = 28).

At 4 weeks of follow-up, remission rates were no different among various active treatment regimens, ranging from 0% to 19% in active treatment arms and 11% for placebo ($P = 0.32$). Response rates were also no different, ranging from 18% to 46% in active treatment arms and 36% in placebo-treated patients ($P = 0.82$). There was no difference in the frequency of adverse events experienced by placebo-treated and repifermin-treated patients.

Colony-stimulating factors

Colony-stimulating factors (CSF) have been considered as potential biological therapies, based upon two observations: (a) a number of genetic syndromes in which there is abnormal neutrophil function (eg, Chediak–Higashi syndrome, chronic granulomatous disease, Hermansky–Pudlak syndrome) have been associated with CD-like GI manifestations, and the efficacy of CSF in managing these patients has been demonstrated; and (b) a case report showing the efficacy of granulocyte (G)-CSF in the treatment of perianal fistula in CD [70].

Pilot studies have suggested that both G-CSF and granulocyte macrophage (GM)-CSF are effective in CD. In CD patients who initially responded to GM-CSF, maintenance treatment with a single daily SC injection of GM-CSF was able to maintain remission at 1-year follow-up [71]. In an 8-week, open-label trial of GM-CSF in patients with active CD, 15 patients were enrolled into one of three treatment groups: 4 µg/kg, 6 µg/kg, or 8 µg/kg [72]. After 8 weeks of treatment, the median response rate was 80%. One patient with a chronic rectovaginal fistula had closure after 3 weeks of treatment.

GM-CSF will require special consideration given its efficacy in treating colitis associated with a number of human genetic syndromes, and, in particular, with regard to fistula closure in patients who have not responded to traditional therapies. Further studies evaluating the role of CSF are anticipated.

Human growth hormone

Human growth hormone (hGH) has been evaluated in the treatment of CD, primarily on the basis of earlier results: animal studies have shown potential for augmenting intestinal epithelial cell growth and human studies, involving patients with short gut syndrome, have shown that hGH improves the tolerability of enteral feeds.

Slonim et al. randomly assigned 37 adults with moderate to severe active CD to 4 months of hGH. The loading dose was 5 mg/day SC for 1 week, followed by a maintenance dose of 1.5 mg/day or placebo [73]. All patients were instructed to undertake a high protein diet. At 4 months of follow-up, there was a significant reduction in CDAI scores among actively treated patients compared with placebo-treated patients (mean 143 ± 44 vs. $19 \pm 63, P = 0.004$).

Additional cytokine-based biological therapies

NF-κB

The NF-κB family of transcriptional regulators represents a critical link in the signal transduction cascade of the GI immune system. Inhibition of this group of proteins might have a significant impact on a whole series of inflammatory mediators.

The 5-aminosalicylate compounds are weak, nonspecific NF-κB inhibitors. In murine models of colitis, enema-based applications of antisense oligonucleotides, targeted to hybridize with NF-κB mRNA, were shown to have some efficacy. This led to a human trial of topical NF-κB antisense oligonucleotides in patients with active distal colonic IBD (CD or UC) [74].

This randomized, placebo-controlled, dose-escalation trial enrolled five patients with UC and six patients with CD. After a single application, clinical responses were noted in 71% of actively treated patients (5/7 patients) compared with 25% in placebo-treated patients (1/4 patients) at 7 days follow-up. Two patients with ulcerative proctitis were in remission beyond 8 and 15 months from treatment. No serious adverse events were noted in this trial.

IFN

IFNs play a significant role in regulating the humoral and cell-mediated immune systems. Recombinant IFN-α has been evaluated in the treatment of both CD and UC. In uncontrolled trials, response rates for CD and UC have ranged upwards of 50% and 93%, respectively [75–78]. Preliminary studies of IFN-β-1a have shown response rates of 50%–80% in both CD and UC patients [79].

A multicenter, Phase 2, randomized, placebo-controlled trial investigated the efficacy of recombinant IFN-α in 97 patients with glucocorticoid-refractory UC [80]. Treatment arms included: 3 million units of SC IFN-α three times weekly (n = 34), 1 million units of IFN-α three times weekly (n = 32), and placebo (n = 31). There was a trend towards significance in remission rates at 8 weeks, with rates of 56%, 38%, and 30%, respectively. Adverse effects including headache, nausea, arthralgia, myalgia, fatigue, and fever were no greater in actively treated patients than placebo-treated patients.

IL-11

The use of rhIL-11 has been evaluated on the basis of its potential role as a protective mediator of the GI mucosal barrier. Data compiled from two clinical trials of rhIL-11 in patients with active CD (N = 264) showed efficacy compared with placebo for

Biological therapy	Administration route	Clinical trials	
		UC	**CD**
TNF-α inhibitors			
Infliximab	IV	X	X
CDP-571	IV	X	X
Etanercept	SC		X
Onercept	SC		X
Thalidomide	PO	X	X
CNI-1493	IV		X
Inhibitors of leukocyte trafficking			
Natalizumab	IV	X	X
LDP-02	IV	X	X
ISIS-2302	IV		X
Inhibitors of Th1 polarization			
IL-10	IV, SC		X
Anti-IFN-α	IV	X	
Anti-IL-2 receptor (daclizumab, basiliximab)	IV	X	
Growth hormones, growth factors, and CSFs			
Epidermal growth factor	PRE	X	
Keratinocyte growth factor	IV	X	
Granulocyte CSF	SC		X
Granulocyte macrophage CSF	SC		X
Human growth hormone	SC		X
Additional cytokine-based biologics			
Antinuclear factor-κB	PRE	X	X
IFN-α	SC	X	X
IFN-β-1a	SC	X	X
IL-11	SC		X

Table 4. Biological therapies evaluated in IBD. CD: Crohn's disease; CSF: colony-stimulating factor; IFN: interferon; IL: interleukin; IV: intravenous; PO: by mouth; PRE: per rectum enema; SC: subcutaneous; Th1: T helper cell type 1; TNF: tumor necrosis factor; UC: ulcerative colitis. X: Clinical trials have taken place.

70. Vaughan D, Drumm B. Treatment of fistulas with granulocyte colony-stimulating factor in a patient with Crohn's disease. *N Engl J Med* 1999;340:239–40.

71. Korzenik J, Pittler A, Dieckgraefe B. Immunostimulation in Crohn's disease: retreatment and maintenance therapy with GM-CSF. *Gastroenterology* 2002;122(4 Suppl. 41):T1204:432A (Abstr.).

72. Dieckgraefe BK, Korzenik JR. Treatment of active Crohn's disease with recombinant human granulocyte-macrophage colony-stimulating factor. *Lancet* 2002;360:1478–80.

73. Slonim AE, Bulone L, Damore MB et al. A preliminary study of growth hormone therapy for Crohn's disease. *N Engl J Med* 2000;342:1633–7.

74. Lofberg R, Neurath M, Ost A et al. Topical NFκB p65 antisense oligonucleotides in patients with active distal colonic IBD. A randomized, controlled, pilot trial. *Gastroenterology* 2002;122(4 Suppl. 41):503A (Abstr.).

75. Hadziselimovic F, Schaub U, Emmons LR. Interferon alpha-2A (roferon) as a treatment of inflammatory bowel disease in children and adolescents. *Adv Exp Med Biol* 1995;371B:1323–6.

76. Sumer N, Palabiyikoglu M. Induction of remission by interferon-alpha in patients with chronic active ulcerative colitis. *Eur J Gastroenterol Hepatol* 1995;7:597–602.

77. Schlichting P, Davidsen B, Madsen SM et al. An open-labeled, randomized study comparing systemic interferon-alpha-2A and prednisolone enemas in the treatment of left-sided ulcerative colitis. *Am J Gastroenterol* 2001;96:1807–15.

78. Gasche C, Reinisch W, Vogelsang H et al. Prospective evaluation of interferon-alpha in treatment of chronic active Crohn's disease. *Dig Dis Sci* 1995;40:800–4.

79. Vantrappen G, Coremans G, Billiau A et al. Treatment of Crohn's disease with interferon. A preliminary clinical trial. *Acta Clin Belg* 1980;35:238–42.

80. Musch E, Raedler A, Andus T et al. A phase II placebo-controlled, randomized, multicenter study to evaluate efficacy and safety of interferon beta-1a in patients with ulcerative colitis. *Gastroenterology* 2002;122(4 Suppl. 41):T1195:431A (Abstr.).

81. Sands BE, Winston BD, Salzberg B et al. Randomized, controlled trial of recombinant human interleukin-11 in patients with active Crohn's disease. *Aliment Pharmacol Ther* 2002;16:399–406.

82. Sands BE, Bank S, Sninsky CA et al. Preliminary evaluation of safety and activity of recombinant human interleukin 11 in patients with active Crohn's disease. *Gastroenterology* 1999;117:58–64.

Serodiagnostics in IBD

Jean-Frédéric Colombel,
Dominique Reumaux, Boualem Sendid,
Patrick Duthilleul, & Daniel Poulain

Introduction

The accuracy of conventional clinical, radiologic, endoscopic, and histologic assessment for the diagnosis of inflammatory bowel disease (IBD) is generally good. Nevertheless, diagnostic dilemmas sometimes persist, and noninvasive, accurate serological assays are still desirable.

Among several serological markers, antineutrophil cytoplasmic antibodies (ANCA) and anti-*Saccharomyces cerevisiae* antibodies (ASCA) have proven to be specific for ulcerative colitis (UC) and Crohn's disease (CD), respectively. Many studies have been conducted within a relatively short period, coinciding with widespread availability of commercial assays. Unfortunately, lack of standardization of the assays has led to controversial results.

This chapter reviews the utility of ANCA and ASCA, and other serological markers, in clinical practice based on recent studies and reviews.

ANCA and ASCA: methodologies

ANCA

ANCA are circulating antibodies that are mainly directed towards constituents of neutrophil granules. ANCA were initially described in primary vasculitides, and subsequently in many inflammatory disorders [1]. In 1990, Saxon et al.

reported the presence of a new subset of ANCA in IBD, and particularly in UC [2].

ANCA are detected using an indirect immunofluorescence (IIF) microscopy assay on ethanol-fixed neutrophils [3]. A sample is considered positive for ANCA when a reaction with neutrophils is observed at a dilution of 1:20. The IIF assay allows semiquantitative evaluation of ANCA titers. Furthermore, it differentiates three main fluorescence patterns [4,5]: cytoplasmic (c)ANCA, perinuclear (p)ANCA, and atypical ANCA patterns.

An International Consensus Statement on Testing and Reporting of ANCA was published in 1999 [6]. In primary vasculitides, the ANCA pattern is cytoplasmic or perinuclear, whereas in IBD, the most frequent pattern is perinuclear, with diffusion towards the cytoplasm. This is variously known as pANCA with diffuse cytoplasmic staining [2], pANCA with "snow drift-like appearance" [7], "x-ANCA" [8], or "atypical ANCA" [9]. According to the International Consensus, the name for these staining patterns should be "atypical ANCA" [6]; nevertheless, in the literature, the ANCA pattern associated with IBD is often termed "pANCA". In clinical practice, a positive IIF test result should always be confirmed by an antigen-specific enzyme-linked immunosorbent assay (ELISA) for proteinase 3-ANCA and myeloperoxidase-ANCA in order to rule out systemic vasculitides [6].

An alterative, three-step procedure (Prometheus Laboratories, Inc., San Diego, California, USA) is used by some investigators.

(a) A fixed neutrophil ELISA is used to screen
     for the presence of ANCA.

(b) IIF staining is then performed on ANCA ELISA-
     positive samples to determine whether a predominantly
     pANCA or cANCA staining pattern is present.

(c) Finally, the specificity of the perinuclear staining pattern is confirmed by its disappearance after deoxyribonuclease (DNase) treatment of the neutrophils.

Results are considered positive when the ANCA titer is above the cut-off (ie, 1/20 dilution) and the IIF reveals perinuclear binding of ANCA that disappears after DNase treatment.

Differences in assay sensitivity and specificity are the most likely explanation for the huge variation in positive results (from 0% to 63%) observed in a population-based study of patients with UC in whom ANCA were screened for by five different laboratories blinded to the diagnosis [10].

ASCA

Using ELISA employing whole killed yeasts cells (ie, *S. cerevisiae* cells) as antigens, elevated anti-*S. cerevisiae* immunoglobulin (Ig)A and IgG levels have been reported in sera from patients with CD, but not in those from patients with UC [11]. This serological response is predominantly directed at sequences of mannose residues expressed in the cell-wall mannan of *S. cerevisiae* [12,13], leading to the designation of ASCA for "anti-*S. cerevisiae* antibodies".

A commercially available ELIASCA test (Diagast, France), based on results obtained by our group [12,14], detects antibodies directed against mannan prepared from *S. cerevisiae* (Su1) grown in bioreactors. Other standardized ASCA kits have also been developed, and some are commercially available. They include antigen derived from disrupted or boiled *S. cerevisiae*, and purified phosphopeptidomannans from the cell wall. Although there is no clear advantage to performing separate testing for IgG and IgA ASCA, most companies provide separate assays [15].

A comparative study of four ASCA tests found a large range of sensitivities and specificities of ASCA for CD, most likely as a consequence of the different cut-off values that were selected for each assay [16].

ANCA and ASCA in the diagnosis of IBD

Keeping methodological variations in mind, ANCA have been detected in the sera of 45%–82% of patients with UC and 2%–28% of patients with CD [17]. Fewer data exist for ASCA, but the prevalences appear more consistent, ranging from 5% to 15% in UC, and from 48% to 69% in CD [17].

Screening for IBD

The clinical value of ANCA or ASCA testing alone in diarrheal diseases is limited by inadequate sensitivity. ANCA positivity has been observed in other colitides, such as eosinophilic and collagenous colitis [18]. The specificity of ASCA seems to be higher, but ASCA positivity has also been observed in patients with celiac disease, primary biliary cirrhosis, and autoimmune hepatitis [19,20]. Thus, the use of serological markers in routine screening for IBD in adults should not be recommended.

The conclusion may be different in children. In a pediatric series, combining the two tests increased the specificity and positive predictive values (PPVs) to 95% and 96%, respectively [21]. As such, these tests could be useful in clinical practice to differentiate between IBD and other diarrheal illnesses. Dubinsky et al. have proposed a sequential diagnostic testing strategy based on serological markers in order to facilitate the diagnosis of IBD in children and to avoid unnecessary evaluations [22].

Screening for indeterminate colitis

Differential diagnosis of CD and UC

The utility of ANCA, ASCA, and their combination in the differential diagnosis of UC and CD is given in **Tables 1** and **2**. The primary test of the diagnostic utility of such markers is to determine whether the PPV (ie, the proportion of patients diagnosed as having CD or UC using serological markers whose true diagnosis was CD or UC) is high enough to be clinically useful. Although arbitrarily fixed, a PPV of at least 85% compared with clinical diagnosis is considered clinically relevant [10]. Taken separately, neither ANCA

Study	Sensitivity (%)		Specificity (%)		PPV (%)	
	ANCA+ for UC	ASCA+ for CD	ANCA+ for UC	ASCA+ for CD	ANCA+ for UC	ASCA+ for CD
Quinton et al. [14]	65	61	85	88	74	**89**
Peeters et al. [53]	50	60	94	86	76	**92**
Koutrobakis et al. [54]	67	39	84	89	**93**	54
Sandborn et al. [10]	63	44	75	87	72	76
Linskens et al. [49]	63	72	86	82	82	80
Ruemmele et al. [21][a]	57	55	92	95	54	**92**
Hoffenberg et al. [55][a]	60	60	65	88	68	80

Table 1. The specificity, sensitivity, and positive predictive value (PPV) of antineutrophil cytoplasmic antibodies (ANCA) for diagnosing ulcerative colitis (UC) and anti-*S. cerevisiae* antibodies (ASCA) for diagnosing Crohn's disease (CD) in patients with inflammatory bowel disease. The numbers in bold represent PPVs >85%. [a]Pediatric population.

nor ASCA consistently meet this outcome for UC or CD (see **Table 1**). However, the combination of ANCA and ASCA assays reached a PPV >85% in four out of five studies (see **Table 2**). Based on these data, clinicians could consider using these combined diagnostic tests as an adjunct to conventional techniques in the differential diagnosis of CD and UC.

All of these studies were retrospective, and all but one [10] were performed in referral center populations, where the patients generally have more severe disease than those seen in general practice. Furthermore, CD patients with different disease locations (ie, small bowel, colon, or both) were included, while the

Study	Sensitivity (%)		Specificity (%)		PPV (%)	
	ANCA+/ ASCA– for UC	ANCA–/ ASCA+ for CD	ANCA+/ ASCA– for UC	ANCA–/ ASCA+ for CD	ANCA+/ ASCA– for UC	ANCA–/ ASCA+ for CD
Quinton et al. [14]	49	57	97	97	**96**	**93**
Peeters et al. [53]	56	44	92	98	**95**	**88**
Koutrobakis et al. [54]	30	58	97	88	77	**93**
Sandborn et al. [10]	38	55	94	81	**86**	75
Linskens et al. [49]	51	64	94	94	**90**	**91**

Table 2. The specificity, sensitivity, and positive predictive value (PPV) of the antineutrophil cytoplasmic antibody (ANCA)/anti-*S. cerevisiae* antibody (ASCA) combination for diagnosing ulcerative colitis (UC) or Crohn's disease (CD) in patients with inflammatory bowel disease. The numbers in bold represent PPVs >85%.

clinical challenge is restricted to patients with pure colitis. A high percentage of CD patients with pure colonic disease and "UC-like" colitis have tested positive for ANCA in some studies [15,23] and, in CD, the presence of ASCA is associated with small-bowel disease [14]. The diagnostic challenge is in patients with pure colitis (ie, to differentiate between colonic CD and UC). Since ASCA are present more frequently in patients with small-bowel disease, they have less relevance in the differential diagnosis of patients with pure colitis.

Serological markers in indeterminate colitis
The results of the first prospective study to assess the usefulness of serological markers in indeterminate colitis (IC) were reported in 2002 [24]. Ninety-seven patients with an initial diagnosis of IC were analyzed for ANCA and ASCA. After a mean follow-up of 1 year, a definitive diagnosis of CD or UC was reached in 31/97

	N (%)	CD (%)	UC (%)	IC (%)
ASCA+/ANCA–	26 (26.8)	8 (30.8)	2 (7.7)	16 (61.5)
ASCA–/ANCA+	20 (20.6)	4 (20)	7 (35)	9 (45)
ASCA+/ANCA+	4 (4.1)	2 (50)	1 (25)	1 (25)
ASCA–/ANCA–	47 (48.5)	3 (6.4)	4 (8.5)	40 (85.1)
Total	97 (100)	17 (17.5)	14 (14.4)	66 (68.1)

Table 3. Diagnostic reliability of antineutrophil cytoplasmic antibodies (ANCA) and anti-*S. cerevisiae* antibodies (ASCA) for diagnosing Crohn's disease (CD) and ulcerative colitis (UC). IC: indeterminate colitis. Reproduced with permission from WB Saunders Co. (*Gastroenterology* 2002;122:1242–7).

(32%) patients (see **Table 3**). ASCA+/ANCA– predicted CD in 80% of IC patients, whereas ASCA–/ANCA+ was predictive for UC in 64% (see **Table 4**) [24]. Nevertheless, 48.5% of IC patients did not have antibodies against ASCA or ANCA (see **Table 3**), thus limiting the clinical utility of serological testing. Interestingly, the majority of these patients remained IC during their further clinical course, perhaps reflecting a distinct clinico-serologic entity.

ANCA and ASCA in disease monitoring

Monitoring disease activity

The relationship between the presence of ANCA and IBD activity remains controversial. Most studies do not support a relationship between the presence or titer of ANCA and UC activity [17]. Hence, in contrast with systemic vasculitides, serial measurement of ANCA titers in IBD is not useful for follow-up of disease activity and prediction of relapses.

The presence of ASCA in CD is stable over time, and is independent of CD activity and duration [14,21,25,26]. The presence of ANCA has been associated with pouchitis after ileal-pouch anastomosis [27,28]. However, most studies were small and retrospective, and contradictory results have been reported [29,30]. In a prospective study, ELISA indicated that

	Diagnosis	Sensitivity (%)	Specificity (%)	PPV (%)	NPV (%)
ASCA+/ ANCA–	CD	8/12 (66.7)	7/9 (77.8)	8/10 (80.0)	7/11 (63.6)
ASCA–/ ANCA+	UC	7/9 (77.8)	8/12 (66.7)	7/11 (63.6)	8/10 (80.0)

Table 4. Sensitivity, specificity, positive predictive value (PPV), and negative predictive value (NPV) of the combination of antineutrophil cytoplasmic antibodies (ANCA) and anti-*S. cerevisiae* antibodies (ASCA) in a prospective study of patients with indeterminate colitis for diagnosing Crohn's disease (CD) and ulcerative colitis (UC). Reproduced with permission from WB Saunders Co. (*Gastroenterology* 2002;122:1242–7).

development of chronic pouchitis was significantly associated with high ANCA levels [31].

Prediction of response to therapy

An attractive field of development for serological markers may be the prediction of response to therapy. The presence of ANCA has been associated with a more refractory type of disease and early requirement for surgery. In a series from the Mayo Clinic, 90% of refractory left-sided UC patients were ANCA-positive versus 62% of patients with treatment-responsive UC ($P = 0.03$) [32].

A higher clinical response to infliximab has been associated with the presence of "speckled" ANCA, defined by the authors as: an ANCA value above the standard assay cut-off, as assessed by ELISA; the absence of distinct pANCA or cANCA staining; and the presence of a diffuse to overtly speckled staining pattern displayed over the entire neutrophil on both the untreated and DNase-treated IIF slides. Lack of response was associated with pANCA [33]. Esters et al. assessed the value of serological markers for prediction of response to infliximab in 279 patients with CD. There was no overall relationship between ASCA or pANCA and response to therapy. However, lower response rates, though not significant, were observed in patients with refractory disease carrying the ANCA+/ASCA– combination

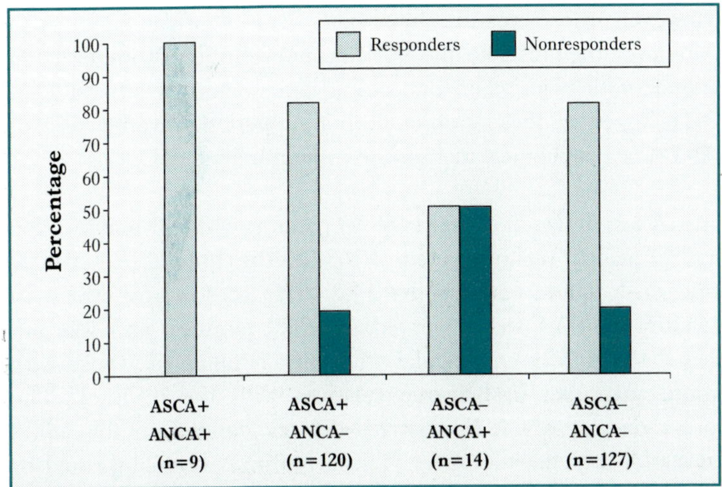

Figure 1. Relationship between the presence or titer of antineutrophil cytoplasmic antibodies (ANCA) and anti-*S. cerevisiae* antibodies (ASCA) and the response to infliximab [34]. Reproduced with permission from Elsevier Science Inc. (*Am J Gastroenterol* 2002;97:1458–62).

(see **Figure 1**) [34]. These observations require confirmation in independent series.

ANCA and ASCA in familial studies

The strongest risk factor for IBD is having a relative with the disease, with a relative risk to siblings of 13–36 for CD and 7–17 for UC [35]. There has been great interest in searching for subclinical markers of IBD in families. Their presence in "unaffected" family members may indicate either a genetic and/or environmental factor predisposing to disease, or identify those in whom an earlier phase of the disease process is occurring.

In 1992, Shanahan et al. found an increased frequency of ANCA in healthy relatives of UC patients compared with controls (16% vs. 3%), with a higher rate of positivity in relatives from ANCA-positive patients [36]. Another family study reported ANCA positivity in 30% of the first-degree relatives of UC patients [37].

However, these results have not been confirmed [38–40]. Moreover, the presence of ANCA was not significantly increased in monozygotic twins where one sibling had UC and the other did not [41]. Together, these studies do not support the hypothesis that ANCA is a subclinical marker for susceptibility to UC.

ASCA was detected in 35/51 (69%) patients with CD and in 13/66 (20%) healthy relatives versus 1/163 healthy controls ($P < 0.0001$ and $P < 0.001$, respectively) [42]. The presence of ASCA in healthy relatives was observed in 12/20 families, and was not restricted to a few particular multiplex families (ie, those with more than two first-degree relatives with the disease). The prevalence of ASCA in relatives did not depend on the ASCA status of affected members. These findings were confirmed by Seibold et al., who found ASCA in 48/193 (25%) healthy first-degree relatives of patients with CD [43].

Conversely, Sutton et al. did not find a significantly increased frequency of ASCA in unaffected relatives (9.3%) of CD patients in comparison with healthy controls (3.8%). However, they demonstrated a high concordance of seropositivity rates in affected family members with seronegative or seropositive probands, and intraclass correlation of quantitative ASCA levels in both affected and unaffected family members [44].

Vermeire et al. studied the prevalence of ANCA and ASCA in a large cohort of patients with sporadic and familial IBD, and their unaffected relatives and spouses (see **Figure 2**) [26]. Overall, ASCA prevalence was the same in both sporadic (63.4%) and familial (62.1%) CD patients. In pure CD families, ASCA were present in 54.2% of CD patients with two affected members versus 74.7% of CD patients with three or more affected members ($P = 0.002$). Of 135 unaffected healthy relatives of CD patients, 28 (20.7%) were ASCA positive.

Interestingly, CD and UC patients in mixed families showed a serological response different from that of sporadic and pure CD

greater for MZ as compared with DZ twins (6% and 0%, respectively) [5].

Ahmad et al. summarized twin studies from three populations [6]. Among 322 twin pairs, net MZ and DZ concordance was, respectively, 37% and 7% for CD, and 10% and 3% for UC. The markedly increased risk for CD in MZ versus DZ twins can only be explained (with the unlikely exception of a shared placental effect) by genetic factors. MZ twin pairs where one twin has UC and the other has CD are extremely rare [7]. This suggests that, in general, specific genetic profiles are required to develop either CD or UC. This strong epidemiologic evidence for the existence of major genetic factors underlying IBD pathogenesis has led investigators to undertake IBD gene discovery research.

Early investigations to identify IBD genes

Initial studies focused on candidate genes – particularly the human leukocyte antigen (HLA) genes – where genetic or protein polymorphisms were known, and where the genes were understood to have a major role in the immune system. For both HLA and non-HLA genes, the most consistent finding from these studies was associations of HLA class II genes (particularly serotype DR2) with UC (see **Table 1**).

Multiple studies reported associations between HLA and CD; however, replication evidence for a specific allele (ie, gene variant) has been more limited. HLA association studies are also complicated because alleles in different genes within the HLA region (also referred to as the major histocompatibility complex [MHC]) are in strong linkage disequilibrium with one another – ie, certain combinations of alleles, located at different sites within the same or proximal genes, have a strong tendency to be inherited together.

For example, both DRB1*1302 (serotype HLA-DR13) and DRB3*0301 (serotype HLA-DR52) have been reported to be

HLA serotype	HLA genotype	Disease	Population	P value[a]	Ref.	Notes
HLA-DR1	DRB1*01	CD	French	0.003 *(Pc)*	8	
	DRB1*0103		Caucasian	0.001	9	
			White, NJ	0.0007	10	Particularly colon-only CD ($P = 0.0002$)
HLA-DR2	DRB1*1502	CD	Japanese	0.0008	11	Inverse association
	DRB1*1501		UK	0.02	12	Inverse association
HLA-DR4	DRB1*0410	CD	Japanese	0.001 *(Pc)*	13	
	DRB1*0401		Caucasian	0.02	14	
HLA-DR7	DRB1*07	CD	French	0.008 *(Pc)*	8	
			German	0.0001	15	
	DRB1*07/		Italy	0.002	16	
	DQB1*0303					
	DRB1*0701		UK	0.04	12	
HLA-DR13	DRB1*1302	CD	Caucasian	0.02	14	
			White, NJ	0.02	17	
HLA-DR52	DRB3*0301	CD	Caucasian	0.0004	14	In LD with DRB*1302
HLA-DR3	DRB1*03	CD	French	< 0.0001 *(Pc)*	8	Inverse association
			German	0.003	15	Inverse association
			Jewish	0.025	17	Inverse association
	DRB1*03/		Italian	0.029	16	Inverse association
	DQB1*0201					

HLA serotype	HLA genotype	Disease	Population	P value[a]	Ref.	Notes
HLA-DQ4	DQB1*04	CD	Japanese	0.001 *(Pc)*	13	
	DQB1*0402	CD	Japanese	0.0001 *(Pc)*	11	
HLA-DR1	DRB1*0103	UC	UK	0.007	18	
			Dutch	0.0002	19	
			UK	0.0001	20	
			Caucasian	0.002	9	Associated with CD in same study
			Mexican	0.001 *(Pc)*	21	
			White, NJ	0.0001	10	Associated with CD in same study
HLA-DR2	NR	UC	Japanese	0.001	22	
	NR		Japanese	0.001	23	
	NR		Japanese	0.008	24	
	NR		Caucasian	0.01	25	pANCA + UC
	DRB1*15		Dutch	0.001	19	
	DRB1*1501		Estonian	0.002	26	pANCA + UC
	DRB1*1502		Japanese	0.0001	27	
			Turkish	0.02	28	
			Japanese	1×10^{-8} *(Pc)*	11	
			Caucasian	0.006	9	Jews and non-Jews, see [25]

Table 1. Human leukocyte antigen (HLA) replicated associations with Crohn's disease (CD) and ulcerative colitis (UC) (positive association unless otherwise noted). DRB3*0301 listed as in strong linkage disequilibrium with DRB1*1302. [a]P value ≤ value given. LD: linkage disequilibrium; NJ: non-Jewish Caucasian; NR: not reported; *Pc*: significance corrected for testing multiple alleles; pANCA + UC: pANCA-positive UC patients.

associated with CD (see **Table 1**), and both are in strong linkage disequilibrium with each other.

Therefore, either genetic variant alone or the combination of both (ie, joint inheritance of both the DRB1*1302–DRB3*0301 alleles together on the same chromosome in the form of a common "haplotype") may be responsible for the observed increased genetic risk for CD. Furthermore, polymorphisms on one HLA gene (eg, HLA class II DR gene) may be in strong linkage disequilibrium with variants on another HLA gene (eg, HLA class II DQ gene) or with variants on other regional genes. For example, DRB1*03 is in strong linkage disequilibrium with tumor necrosis factor (TNF)-α promoter polymorphism –308*2 [29].

The multitude of positive association studies in the HLA region suggest that one or more genes in the region have allelic variants that may alter gene function and thereby increase the risk of developing IBD. Common patterns of association are beginning to appear. However, no study has thus far been able to discern which single gene variant within the HLA region, above all other gene polymorphisms, is the biologically causative variant.

Studies that have examined potential associations of polymorphisms in non-HLA genes with IBD have shown both positive and negative findings [30,31]. Most of the positive findings have not been replicated, and even for those positive studies with some replications (eg, interleukin 1 receptor antagonist [IL-1RN] and UC), the associations are still not considered established – or, as we will show with intracellular adhesion molecule (ICAM)-1, different alleles have been associated in different studies.

There have been numerous candidate gene studies published in the past 2 years. These will be explored in detail in the latter part of this chapter.

Genome screens to identify regions of human chromosomes containing IBD genes: the first IBD genetic locus (IBD1) and the discovery of the *NOD2* gene

The identification of repetitive sequences (particularly dinucleotide, trinucleotide, and tetranucleotide "microsatellite" repeat markers) spread throughout the human genome and high-throughput genotyping methods have allowed IBD genetics investigators, beginning in 1996, to perform whole-genome linkage studies in families with multiple persons affected with IBD (ie, "multiplex" families).

These studies identified regions of chromosomes ("genetic loci") that had evidence for encoding susceptibility genes for IBD [32]. There are seven defined IBD chromosomal loci (IBD1–IBD7) with either genome-wide linkage evidence (ie, 5% error per whole-genome analysis or logarithm of the odds [LOD] of linkage >3.3 or $P < 2\times10^{-5}$ [33]) or strong replication of linkage evidence (see **Table 2**). Other chromosomal regions that have demonstrated linkage evidence (but not genome-wide) in more than one report are 3p, 4q, and 7q.

Among the IBD loci identified, IBD1 is unique. Following the initial identification of a chromosome 16, IBD1 CD locus by Hugot et al. in 1996 [34], there has been replication evidence for IBD1 in seven other independent studies [35–40,42]. Such consistent linkage evidence for a common complex genetic disorder in a non-HLA locus was remarkable; this degree of consistency had not been found for any other non-HLA loci for common autoimmune complex genetic disorders (eg, type 1 diabetes or rheumatoid arthritis).

Table 2 lists chromosomal regions with nominal ($P \leq 0.01$) or greater linkage evidence in a genome screen and evidence of replication in one or more reports. The IBD1–IBD7 loci have all

Locus	Chromosomal location	Initial report	Replications/extension	Disease
IBD1	Pericentromeric 16	Hugot, 1996 [34][a]	Ohmen, 1996 [35] Parkes, 1996 [36] Brant, 1998 [37] Curran, 1998 [38] Cavanaugh, 1998 [39] Annesse, 1999 [40] (Brant, 2000 [41])[a,b] Akolkar, 2001 [42][c] (Cavanaugh, 2001 [43])[a]	CD
IBD2	12p13.2–q24.1	Satsangi, 1996 [44][a]	Duerr, 1998 [45] Curran, 1998 [38] Yang, 1999 [46] (Parkes, 2000 [47])[d] (Cavanaugh, 2001 [43])	IBD; UC>CD
IBD3	6p21–p23	Hampe, 1999 [56]	Yang, 1999 [48] (Hampe, 1999 [49])[a] Rioux, 2000 [50] Dechairo, 2001 [51] (Fisher, 2002 [52])[e]	IBD
IBD4	14q11–q12	Ma, 1999 [53]	Duerr, 2000 [54][a]	CD
IBD5	5q31	Rioux, 2000 [50][a]		CD

Locus	Chromosomal location	Initial report	Replications/extension	Disease
IBD6	19p13	Cho, 1998 [55]	Duerr, 2000 [54] Rioux, 2000 [50][a]	CD
IBD7	1p36	Cho, 1998 [55]	Hampe, 1999 [56] (Cho, 2000 [57]) Paavola, 2001 [58]	IBD
–	3p25–p21	Satsangi, 1996 [44]	Rioux, 2000 [50] Hampe, 2001 [60] Paavola, 2001 [58] Duerr, 2002 [59][g]	IBD
–	4q22–q26	Cho, 1998 [55]	Hampe, 1999 [56]	IBD/UC
–	7p13-q21	Satsangi, 1996 [44]	Cho, 1998 [55]	IBD

Table 2. IBD genetic loci with genome-wide significance or replications. Replications are limited to reports with significant evidence for replication ($P \leq 0.01$). Reports in parentheses include pedigrees genotyped by the same authors with evidence for the same locus in an earlier report. [a]Individual study with genome-wide linkage evidence. [b]Includes pedigrees from Brant et al. [37], significance genome-wide (LOD 3.84, not corrected for multiple testing) in a subset of Crohn's disease (CD) pedigrees with early-onset and more severe CD. [c]Replication evidence significant for the subset of pedigrees with early-onset CD. [d]Data compiled from previous Satsangi et al. and Duerr et al. genome-wide screens showing evidence in ulcerative colitis (UC) pedigrees. [e]Male-specific linkage evidence, data from Hampe 1999 [56]. [f]Haplotype <1 cM identified in unrelated Chaldean IBD families. [g]Evidence at 3p26. IBD: inflammatory bowel disease.

had genome-wide evidence in one study or equivalent evidence from two or more studies combined. Loci other than IBD1 with several replications include IBD2 on chromosome 12 [44] and IBD3 [56], which overlaps the HLA region, on chromosome 6p (see **Table 2**).

Proof of the IBD1 locus

The International IBD Genetics Consortium undertook the challenge to assemble an IBD multiplex pedigree cohort large enough to have power to assess the validity of different IBD loci and narrow the size of loci intervals.

Twelve IBD genetic research centers from six countries assembled DNA samples from 613 Caucasian families containing at least two siblings with IBD [43]. These samples were genotyped with a panel of 12 genetic markers that spanned the chromosome 16/IBD1 and chromosome 12/IBD2 loci.

For the 386 CD-only pedigrees, there was conclusive evidence for a CD locus on chromosome 16q12.1 (multipoint maximum LOD score [MLS] 5.79) [43]. These CD pedigrees did not include those that Hugot et al. had used to initially identify the IBD1/chromosome 16 locus [34]. Evidence for linkage was equally strong in Jewish and non-Jewish CD families. There was no evidence for linkage among the UC families (n = 108) or "mixed" families (ie, those with both UC and CD; n = 119) .

NOD2: an IBD1 causative gene

IBD genetics investigators used two strategies to identify an IBD1 gene. One strategy was to identify specific genetic variants (ie, alleles of microsatellite or single nucleotide polymorphism [SNP] markers) located within the pericentromeric chromosome 16 region that were in linkage disequilibrium (ie, inherited together) with the CD phenotype.

Association was primarily tested by the transmission/ disequilibrium test (TDT) [61]. The TDT examines whether a specific allele, observed in heterozygous parents, is transmitted to their affected offspring at a rate significantly greater than 50%. Fifty percent is the expected transmission of any given marker or gene allele in a heterozygous parent, as predicted by Mendel's law of independent assortment. Greater than 50% transmission of an allele to offspring indicates that transmission of the allele is not independent of phenotype; therefore, the allele is associated with CD. TDT has an advantage over the more common case-control association test (ie, determining if an allele is more frequent in the CD cases as compared with ethnically matched controls) in that TDT cannot be confounded by unrecognized population stratification between cases and controls [30].

Hugot et al. used the TDT to test parent/CD-child "trio" pedigrees for association with microsatellite markers that span the pericentromeric region of chromosome 16 [62]. CD was strongly associated with two alleles of the genetic marker D16S3136 in two independent sets of CD trios. D16S3136, located only 2 cM telomeric of the International Consortium chromosome 16 peak, mapped within the middle of a novel gene; alleles of several SNPs located on this gene's exons were also in strong linkage disequilibrium with CD. That gene was *NOD2*, a gene that Gabriel Nunez's group at the University of Michigan had concurrently identified based on *NOD2*'s homology (39%) to the *NOD1* gene that they had previously described [63].

NOD proteins

NOD (nucleotide-binding oligomerization domain) proteins are intracellular proteins that function as part of the innate immune system. They regulate apoptosis and serve as signal transducers for bacterial lipopolysaccharides (LPS) via transcription activation of inflammatory pathways mediated by nuclear factor (NF)-κB. NOD proteins contain three elements:

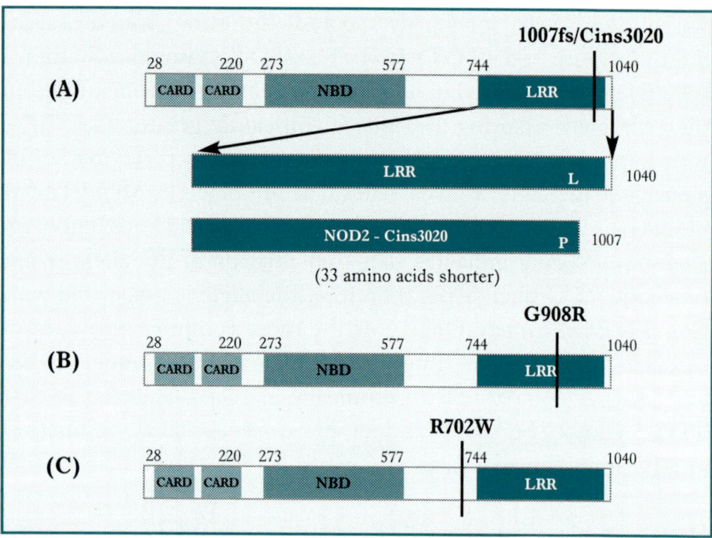

Figure 2. Schematic diagram of NOD2 protein structure (bars). The numbers above the bars represent amino acids from the N-terminus. The vertical lines extending through the protein diagrams indicate: **(A)** a C-nucleotide insertion at coding nucleotide 3020, resulting in a leucine to proline substitution at amino acid 1007, and a stop codon causing the 33-amino acid deletion; **(B)** a G to C nucleotide mutation at coding nucleotide 2722, resulting in a glycine to arginine missense mutation at amino acid 908 in the leucine repeat region (LRR); **(C)** a C to T nucleotide mutation at coding nucleotide 2104, resulting in an arginine to tryptophan missense mutation at amino acid 702. CARD: caspase-recruitment domain; NBD: nucleotide-binding domain.

- N-terminal, caspase recruitment domain(s) (known as CARD), which function in apoptosis regulation

- a centrally located nucleotide-binding domain (NBD)

- a C-terminal leucine-rich repeat region (LRR) (see **Figure 2**)

The LRR domains of NOD proteins bind various bacterial LPS and peptidoglycans. The N-terminal CARD interacts with the CARD of the protein RIP-like interacting CLARP kinase (RICK).

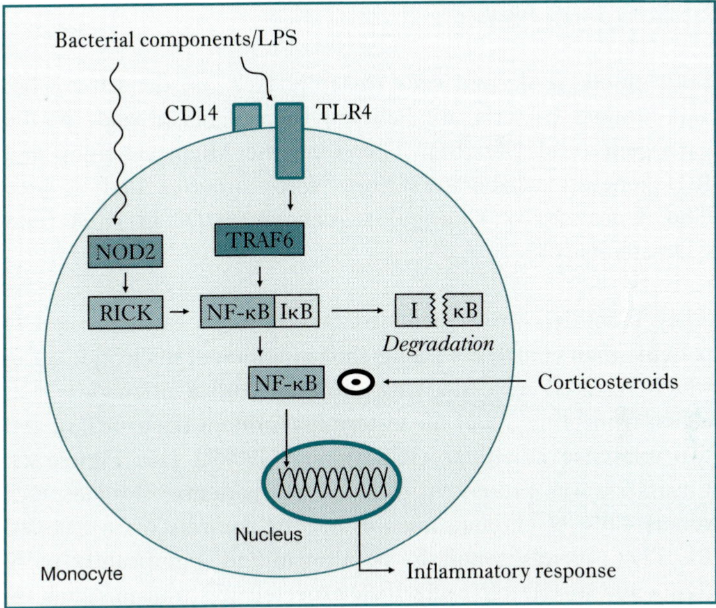

Figure 3. Outline of the innate immune response to bacterial components. IκB: inhibitor of NF-κB; LPS: lipopolysaccharide; NF: nuclear factor; RICK: RIP-like interacting CLARP kinase; TRAF: tumor necrosis factor receptor-associated factor. Reproduced with permission from the Lancet Publishing Group (*Lancet* 2001;357:1902–4).

RICK causes inhibitor of NF-κB (IκB) to dissociate from the NF-κB/IκB complex, causing release of active NF-κB (see **Figure 3**).

NOD2 made an ideal candidate for a CD susceptibility gene for the following reasons:

- it mapped to the peak IBD1 linkage region

- its expression appeared to be primarily in cells of the monocyte lineage

- it acts as a bacterial LPS receptor to activate the major transcription regulator of inflammation, NF-κB

Sequencing *NOD2*

Both monocyte-derived cells (macrophages and dendritic cells) and luminal bacteria are believed to play major roles in the pathogenesis of CD [64]. Therefore, the Michigan group and IBD genetics collaborators from North America (led by Judy Cho, University of Chicago) sequenced *NOD2* in DNA from CD patients [65].

They identified three major mutations more common in CD patients than controls: a frame-shift mutation at nucleotide 3020, which resulted in a missense mutation and a premature stop codon truncating 3% of the C-terminal protein (Leu1007fs); and two missense mutations (R702W and G908R) (see **Figure 2**). Leu1007fs was present in 8.2% of CD patients' chromosomes versus 4.0% of chromosomes of healthy controls ($P = 0.0018$). By TDT, it was found to be transmitted significantly more frequently to CD offspring than expected (39 transmissions vs. 17 nontransmissions, $P = 0.0046$).

Independently, Hugot et al. similarly sequenced the *NOD2* putative exons among their collection of western European CD patients [62]. Twenty-nine percent of CD patients' chromosomes contained one of the three major *NOD2* mutations as compared with 7% of controls' chromosomes. CD patients were three times as likely to carry a single *NOD2* mutation ("mutant heterozygotes") as healthy controls. More striking was that CD patients were 38–44 times more likely to carry two *NOD2* mutations – whether the same mutation ("simple homozygotes") or two different mutations ("compound homozygotes") – than healthy controls. Thus, the risk of *NOD2* mutant alleles causing CD has a strong recessive component – consistent with estimates of CD inheritance from segregation analyses [66].

Hugot et al. also identified multiple rare *NOD2* coding mutations in CD patients [62,67]. The relatively high frequency of the frame-shift mutation in the control population (9% of healthy people were heterozygote carriers) and the presence of multiple additional amino acid-altering variants suggest that *NOD2* mutations arose from a historical selection pressure; at some point in history, carrying *NOD2* mutations may have yielded a survival advantage.

Functional studies of NOD2

In addition to powerful genetic evidence that *NOD2* is a major risk factor for CD, *in vitro* functional studies show that the Leu1007fs mutant does not function properly as a bacterial LPS regulator of inflammation [65]. As compared with wild-type *NOD2* constructs, Leu1007fs mutant expression constructs transfected into human embryonic kidney HEK293T cells fail to activate NF-κB in response to bacterial LPS. Very recently, both the R702W and the G908R NOD2 mutant proteins were shown *in vitro* to produce only weak activation of NF-κB (as compared with wild-type NOD2) in response to bacterial LPS or peptidoglycan [68].

These results were surprising, as they appeared to contradict the notion that CD is associated with up-regulated NF-κB activity [69]. There are several hypotheses to explain these seemingly paradoxical findings within the context of CD pathophysiology, including: (a) failure of *NOD2* mutant monocytes or macrophages to sense bacteria may result in an aggravated response by the adaptive immune system [65]; (b) some NF-κB isoforms may be inhibitory, notably p50 homodimers [70]; (c) the altered LRR of mutant NOD2 proteins may be hyperresponsive to certain uncharacterized bacterial LPS. Caution must be exercised in interpreting these initial results [65,68]; these studies were performed *in vitro* and in nonmonocytic cell lines.

NOD2 as a risk factor for CD

Despite our lack of understanding of how mutant *NOD2* causes risk for CD, its discovery has further established certain long-held etiopathogenic assumptions about CD:

- CD, at least in some individuals, has a definite genetic basis

- some individuals who are susceptible to CD (ie, those with *NOD2* mutations) have a genetically disordered immune system

- monocytes and their lineages play a major role in CD pathophysiology

- in CD patients, the immune response to bacteria is abnormal

NOD2 is an established risk factor for CD. The initial reports by Ogura et al. [65] and Hugot et al. [62] have been replicated several times; without exception, all reports found *NOD2* mutations to be increased in CD patients (see **Table 3**).

It is important to note that though *NOD2* carriers of two mutant alleles have up to 40 times the population risk for CD, the estimated penetrance of even these relatively high-risk *NOD2* homozygotes and compound heterozygotes is likely no greater than 3% or 4% [62,76]. Because only 8%–17% (the latter figure includes the rare mutations observed by Lesage et al. [67]) of CD patients are homozygous or compound heterozygous for *NOD2* [12,62,67,71,75], overall, less than two in every 10,000 people will have CD and be *NOD2* homozygotes or compound heterozygotes (assuming a CD population prevalence of 0.1%).

In comparison, based on *NOD2* mutation allele frequency in healthy controls [12,62,67,71–73], the overall population frequency of *NOD2* homozygotes/compound heterozygotes is estimated to be 36–100 per 10,000 people. Thus, less than two out of these 36–100 people, or roughly 2%–5%, are likely to develop CD. Obviously, well-controlled population studies need to be performed to clarify these grossly estimated risks.

NOD2 can only account for a small proportion of the overall CD familial genetic risk, and the attributable risk is estimated at

Ref.	Population	CD cases	CD allele frequency	Control allele frequency	Family history of IBD	Younger age at diagnosis	Any ileal disease	Stricturing	Fistulizing	Surgery
67	W Europe	453	0.33	0.10	NS	+		+	NS	NS
12	UK	244	0.26	0.08		+	+	NS	NS	NS
71	NW Europe	560	0.22	0.07	+		+			
72	Germany[a]	550	0.31	0.10			+			
73	Quebec	231	0.28	0.06	NS	NS	+	NS	NS	+
74	US	142				NS		+	NS	NS
75	US	275	0.26	0.10	NS	+[b]	+	+	+[c]	NS

Table 3. Phenotype features more frequent among Crohn's disease (CD) patients with *NOD2* mutations than among CD patients without *NOD2* mutations. [a]Phenotype results for 444 retrospective German cases, confirmed in 106 prospective cases. [b]After correcting for attained age at diagnosis. [c]Nonperianal fistulizing. "All fistulizing disease" (perianal and nonperianal) was not significant in any study. NW Europe: north-western Europe (UK, Germany, and The Netherlands) patients and controls. NS: nonsignificant. +: phenotype found significantly more frequently ($P < 0.05$) in either carriers of any *NOD2* mutations or more frequent only in CD patients who are carriers of two *NOD2* mutant alleles (simple homozygotes or compound heterozygotes) than in patients with no *NOD2* mutations (wild-type homozygotes).

<25% [62]. Therefore, other IBD susceptibility genes must interact with *NOD2* to cause CD risk. Investigators are now reanalyzing their linkage studies to determine the presence of epistatic interactions between some of the identified IBD loci and *NOD2*. Stratifying linkage results based on *NOD2* mutation status may help to identify those gene regions which contain *NOD2*-interactive IBD-susceptibility genes.

How *NOD2* has advanced our understanding of CD

NOD2 may explain ethnic differences in CD incidence. The prevalence of CD in Asian populations is consistently less than that in western European populations. However, it has been uncertain if this difference is genetic or geographic. The *NOD2* gene mutations provide a solid foundation to examine genetic differences in IBD etiology by ethnicity.

In patients of Japanese ancestry, Inoue et al. found none of the three common *NOD2* mutations in 350 CD patients, 272 UC patients, or 292 healthy controls [77]. Moreover, Yamazaki et al. also found none of the three common *NOD2* mutations in 483 Japanese CD patients [78]. One patient did contain a novel polymorphism (R702Q), but there were no novel *NOD2* amino acid changes in the LRR region sequenced. Similarly, Croucher et al. recently reported finding no *NOD2* mutant alleles or haplotypes in 126 Korean CD patients or in 116 Korean controls [79].

CD prevalence in Ashkenazi Jews is consistently greater than that in non-Jews [80]. The Leu1007fs mutant allele was found to be equally present in Ashkenazi Jews and non-Jewish Caucasians [65]. However, the G908R mutant allele was found to be more than twice as common in Ashkenazim than non-Jewish whites (allele frequency: 8.7% Ashkenazim CD vs. 4.3% non-Jewish CD) [68]. Conversely, the R702W mutant allele is relatively rare in CD in Ashkenazim as compared with CD in non-Jewish whites (2.6% vs. 10.8%, respectively) [68].

NOD2 and CD clinical heterogeneity

In part, *NOD2* explains CD clinical heterogeneity. In 2000, we reported that IBD1 linkage evidence was found almost entirely in CD families with no history of UC, early age at onset, and a history of more severe disease, as noted by a history of bowel resection surgery or use of immunomodulators such as 6-mercaptopurine, azathioprine, or methotrexate [41]. This suggested that the IBD1 gene may also influence CD phenotypic expression.

Multiple *NOD2* phenotype studies have reported remarkably consistent results (see **Table 3**). The main findings are as follows.

- *NOD2* is a significant risk factor for people both with and without a family history of IBD. This demonstrates that genetic risk for CD exists in both familial and sporadic cases. Most studies found similar *NOD2* mutant allele frequencies in familial versus nonfamilial CD [67,73,75]. However, two studies did find that *NOD2* mutations were even more frequent in familial versus nonfamilial CD [71,81]; most notably, Zhou et al. recently observed a marked increased frequency of *NOD2* G908R mutations in Ashkenazim familial versus sporadic CD (0.127 vs. 0.059, respectively) [81].

- *NOD2* is a CD – but not a UC – risk gene. In fact, *NOD2* mutations may be slightly less common in UC patients than in healthy controls [67,76].

- *NOD2* carriers with CD, particularly homozygotes or compound heterozygotes, have ileal or ileal–colonic CD, and only rarely have colonic-only CD. This is a major phenotypic observation associated with *NOD2*. This is also consistent with the relatively low frequency of *NOD2* mutations in UC. These observations suggest that CD involving the ileum may be etiologically distinct from CD restricted to the colon [12,71–73,75].

- In multiple studies, *NOD2* mutations have been associated with stricturing CD, particularly for persons carrying two mutations. *NOD2*'s association with stricturing CD is independent of its risk for ileal involvement [67,74,75].

- Consistent with linkage studies [41,42], *NOD2* is more associated with early-onset than later-onset CD [12,67,75].

Two studies have shown a trend [67,75], and one showed significance [73], for an association of *NOD2* mutations with a history of surgical resection. This trend may be explained by the association of *NOD2* with ileal disease: in patients with ileal disease involvement, we observed no differences in surgical-free survival resection between *NOD2* mutation carriers and *NOD2* wild-type patients [75].

NOD2 and response to therapy

An area of great anticipation for clinicians is whether *NOD2* mutations can predict response to medication therapy. The association of *NOD2* with stricturing complications suggests that *NOD2* carriers should be closely observed for the development of stricturing symptoms and treated judiciously. *NOD2* double mutants should also be closely evaluated for the presence of ileal disease, even if their clinical symptoms suggest only colonic CD.

Two studies have evaluated *NOD2* with respect to response to anti-TNF-α antibody therapy (infliximab) [82,83]; neither found any association. This may not be surprising, as infliximab is particularly effective in the treatment of perianal fistulae, and there appears to be a slight inverse association between *NOD2* mutations and the presence of perianal fistulae [12]. Studies of patients' responses to other medications, such as 6-mercaptopurine, in relation to *NOD2* mutation status are greatly anticipated.

Unique *NOD2* mutations and Blau syndrome

A unique set of *NOD2* mutations – those in the nucleotide-binding domain (R334L, R334Q, R334W, and L469F) – are present in families with the multiple granulomatous autosomal dominant disorder Blau syndrome [84,85]. These mutations have not been observed in CD patients. Interestingly, patients with Blau syndrome have uveitis, granulomatous arthritis, and skin lesions (ie, the common extraintestinal granuloma sites in CD), but they do not develop intestinal granulomas.

Evidence for IBD1 genes other than *NOD2*

Hampe et al. found that *NOD2* mutations can only account for a portion of the pericentromeric chromosome 16 linkage evidence [86]. In a study of German and British (UK) IBD patients, Hampe et al. reported the presence of a risk haplotype 20 cM p-telomeric of *NOD2*, on the pericentromeric p-arm of chromosome 16 at marker D16S3068 [86].

There was significant evidence for this haplotype in the German subset of pedigrees, particularly in those persons with IBD who did not carry the major *NOD2* mutations (ie, in their population R702W or Leu1007fs). In the UK patients, evidence was weak – but present – in the immediately adjacent genetic markers. This pericentromeric 16p region should be considered "interesting" and further studied for replication. No known genes were described within the immediate region of the haplotype [86].

IBD2/chromosome 12 locus

In the International IBD Genetics Consortium IBD multiplex pedigree cohort, only weak evidence was found for IBD2 among 89 UC families (MLS 1.2), and there was no significant evidence for IBD2 among 349 CD or 545 all-IBD pedigrees (CD and mixed pedigrees) [43]. Greatest linkage evidence was observed at the more q-centromeric chromosome 12q markers genotyped in the study (D12S85 and D12S368). An Oxford University/University of Pittsburgh study found similar support for IBD2 being primarily a UC locus [47]. These studies suggest that further research is needed in larger samples of UC patients to define the IBD2 locus on chromosome 12.

IBD3/chromosome 6p locus

The German/UK and Canadian IBD genome-wide screens found evidence suggestive of linkage for chromosome 6p (LOD scores of 2.1 and 2.3, respectively), overlapping the HLA region [50,56].

In a follow-up investigation [49], the German/UK IBD genetics group expanded their study population from 268 to 339 pedigrees and genotyped an additional 11 microsatellite markers across the HLA region. They found significant evidence of linkage, maximum at marker D6S461 (MLS 4.2), in the total set of IBD pedigrees (ie, CD, UC, and mixed) [49]. This peak linkage evidence was 3 cM p-telomeric of the TNF-α gene. Evidence for transmission disequilibrium (by TDT) was reported for marker D6S426 ($P = 0.004$), 20 cM centromeric of the peak. To be considered compelling, either this finding needs to be replicated, or alleles on other markers in the immediate region must also be shown to be over-transmitted and exist on a common risk haplotype.

Yang et al. found significant evidence of linkage for TNF microsatellite markers by using haplotype-sharing analyses in siblings concordant for CD versus siblings discordant for CD [48]. This study demonstrated that linkage to the HLA region is present in CD-only sibling pairs (by linear regression analysis, $P = 3 \times 10^{-5}$).

Dechairo et al. [51] studied 234 IBD pedigrees that included the Oxford University, UK genome-screen cohort [44] (see "Linkage on other chromsomes" below). They genotyped 11 markers spanning 75 cM across the chromosome 6p region. Linkage evidence was maximum at D6S291 (MLS 3.04), 13 cM centromeric to the TNF-α region. However, the marker density in this region was only 10 cM, and thus too small to localize IBD3 with accuracy. Linkage evidence was equivalent in CD and UC pedigrees.

Recently, the German/UK IBD Genetics Group reanalyzed their genome-wide screen, and performed sex-stratified analyses in families containing male-only or female-only members with IBD [52]. The maximum MLS occurred at D6S291 (the same peak marker in the Dechairo et al. study, above), with a male MLS of 5.91 versus a female MLS of 0.06. There was also evidence for sex-specific linkage in males on chromosomes 11 and 14; however, these regions did not overlap previously identified IBD loci.

The authors noted that sex differences in HLA haplotype frequencies have been reported in other immune-mediated diseases, notably type 1 diabetes, multiple sclerosis, and rheumatoid arthritis. They did not observe sex-specific linkage for the IBD1/chromosome 16 region.

A recently published genome-wide screen evaluated linkage in 63 IBD pedigrees containing 117 affected relative pairs from Nova Scotia [87]. A 12 cM density marker set was used, the same as in the Rioux et al. Canadian screen [50]. A novel locus on chromosome 11p15 was observed (nonparametric linkage score 2.3, $P = 0.014$) with suggestive evidence of linkage (one false-positive per three genome screens [33]) by simulation analyses [87]. There was weak evidence to replicate IBD3 and IBD1.

Interestingly, the authors performed a meta-analysis of their new IBD genome-wide screen and four prior published genome-wide screens [50,53,55,56] using the genome search meta-analysis method of Wise et al [88]. For every genome screen, each 30 cM region or "bin" of the genome (excluding chromosome X) was ranked, from the region with greatest evidence for linkage (rank #1) to the region with the lowest evidence for linkage (rank #117). The rankings for all bins were then averaged to find the regions with the greatest average (or weighted average) linkage evidence.

For both IBD ($P = 0.000087$) and CD ($P = 0.0013$), the IBD3/HLA region had by far the greatest average evidence for linkage by this method, using both average and weighted average methods, although in none of these individual genome screens was IBD3 the one locus with greatest linkage evidence! Less significant, even for CD, were the IBD1 and IBD5 regions. Therefore, IBD3 appears to be the most consistent locus, although its influence is relatively moderate.

IBD5/chromosome 5q locus

An important development in IBD genetics was the identification of a definitive CD locus in the cytokine cluster of chromosome 5q. In a genome-wide screen of Canadian IBD pedigrees, IBD genetics investigators found genome-wide evidence for CD loci on chromosomes 5q and 19p [50].

Peak linkage evidence for the 5q locus was within a cytokine-rich region that contains genes encoding interleukin (IL)-3, IL-4, IL-5, IL-13, interferon (IFN) regulatory factor 1, and the polyhydroxylase gene, *P4HA2*. This region has also been associated with asthma [89]. Using a strategy of overlapping TDT linkage disequilibrium analyses, the same investigators identified a chromosomal region spanning 600,000 bp that was tightly associated with CD in 420 unrelated pedigrees (both with and without a CD family history) [90].

They screened the 11 genes that mapped between IL-4 and IL-3 for mutations. This screen included those genes described above. However, they identified no apparent functional polymorphisms or mutations. Four major haplotypes were identified within this region, one of which was closely associated with CD. Risk of CD was increased 2-fold for persons carrying one risk haplotype and 6-fold for those carrying two risk haplotypes.

Future strategies to identify the actual disease polymorphisms within this region will include identification of all the genes encoded within the minimal risk haplotype, extensive screening for mutations/polymorphisms in additional subjects that carry the risk haplotype, and perhaps linkage disequilibrium mapping studies in more genetically diverse populations – such as African Americans – to potentially further narrow the risk region.

5q31 candidate genes: IL-4 and monocyte differentiation antigen CD14
IL-4 maps to the cytokine region of the IBD5 CD locus at 5q31. It is secreted by T-helper type 2 lymphocytes and mediates the humoral immune response. Two studies found an association of promoter polymorphisms of IL-4 with CD, but not UC [91,92]. However, the variants associated with CD in each study were different (see **Table 4)**. The (–590)T allele has previously been associated with atopy. Both studies also looked for associations of the IL-4 receptor, located on chromosome 16 p-centromeric IBD1 region, with CD. There was no evidence that the IL-4 receptor (see **Table 4**) had an independent association with CD, though the Aithal et al. report indicated a potential interaction of the IL-4 receptor variant Q576R and IL-4 promoter polymorphism allele (–34T), resulting in CD risk [92].

The monocyte antigen CD14 is critical for LPS-dependent signal transduction and maps to 5q31. It also interacts with inflammatory infectious diseases to enhance the production of several proinflammatory cytokines, such as IL-1, IL-6, TNF-α, and IFN-γ. CD14 also maps to the 5q31 candidate region. The functional CD14 promoter polymorphism (–159 T/C) has been described, and TT homozygotes showed significantly higher serum levels of soluble CD14 [105].

Klein et al. studied 219 CD patients, 142 UC patients, and 410 controls, and found that the T allele and TT genotype were associated with CD, but not UC [105]. In contrast, an IBD study in the Japanese population (82 CD, 101 UC, 123 controls) reported that the T allele and TT genotypes were associated with UC, but not CD [104]. It remains to be investigated as to whether or not the associations reported for IL-4 and CD14 are independent of the IBD5 Canadian risk haplotype [90].

Linkage on other chromosomes
In the initial Oxford genome screen, two IBD loci were identified on chromosomes 3p and 7q, with evidence suggestive of linkage [44]. Using a dense set of markers (mapping density <2 cM) that

Ref.	Association	Locus	Chromosome	Gene/polymorphism	Samples tested	Findings	Ethnicity
93			1q31	IL-10 (−627, −1117)	90 CD, 159 UC, 227 controls	No IBD associations	UK
94	+		2q14	IL-1RN*2	910 UC, 1925 controls	Meta-analysis: IL-1RN*2; allele frequency ($P = 0.01$)	European
95				IL-1RN*2, IL-1B	182 CD, 347 UC, 289 controls	No IBD or UC associations	Caucasian
96	+			IL-1RN*1	218 CD, 124 UC, 401 controls	IL1RN*1; inverse with IBD, particularly CD ($P = 0.048$)	Belgium
97			2q33	CTLA4 (C −318T, A +49G)	163 CD, 139 UC, 174 controls/35 UC, 62 controls	No IBD associations	Dutch/Chinese
98	+		2q35	NRAMP1 promoter	117 CD, 98 UC, 324 controls	Allele 7 frequency increased in CD ($Pc = 0.015$) and UC ($Pc = 0.018$)	Japanese
99	+		3p21	MLH1, D3S1768, D3S1611	52 CD, 60 UC, 51 controls	Association of two MLH1 microsatellites and CD	Italy
100				CCR5Δ32	538 IBD, 135 controls	No IBD associations	Belgian
101					235 CD, 346 controls	No CD associations	German
58					16 CD, 71 UC, 37 mixed sibpairs	No IBD associations	Finnish
102					99 CD, 251 UC, 103 controls	No IBD associations	NE England
60					162 CD, 114 UC, 77 mixed sibpairs	No IBD associations	UK/German

Ref.	Association	Locus	Chromosome	Gene/polymorphism	Samples tested	Findings	Ethnicity
60			3p21	CCR2 (Ile64Val)	162 CD,114 UC, 77 mixed sibpairs	No IBD associations	UK/German
101					235 CD, 346 controls	No CD associations	German
60			3p26	IL–5RA	162 CD, 114 UC, 77 mixed sibpairs	No IBD associations	UK/German
103			5q21	APC (I1307K)	306 IBD (211 CD, 86 UC), 308 unaffecteds	No IBD associations	Ashkenazim
91	+	IBD5	5q31	IL–4 (–590T)	221 CD, 147 UC, 446 controls	(–590T) inverse with CD ($P = 0.03$), IL–4RA; no IBD associations	German
92	+			IL–4 (–34T)	86 CD, 98 UC, 321 controls	IL–4 (–34T) and CD ($P = 0.002$), association IL–4RA(Q576R) in CD ($P = 0.09$)	UK
104	+			CD14 (–159T/C)	82 CD, 101 UC, 123 controls	T allele ($P = 0.0074$) and T/T genotype ($P = 0.022$) in UC, not in CD	Japanese
105	+				219 CD, 142 UC, 410 controls	T allele ($P = 0.044$) and T/T genotype ($P = 0.005$) in CD, not in UC	German
106		IBD3	6p21.3	MICA, MICB (5, 13 variants)	94 CD, 94 UC, 154 controls	No IBD associations	Caucasian
107				MICA, MICB (46, 17 variants)	248 CD, 329 UC, 354 controls	No significant IBD associations (corrected for multiple testing)	UK

Ref.	Association	Locus	Chromosome	Gene/polymorphism	Samples tested	Findings	Ethnicity
108	+	IBD3	6p21.3	MICA A6 allele	83 UC, 132 controls	Association UC by allele frequency: ($Pc = 0.000011$) early onset homozygotes ($Pc = 0.0042$)	Japanese
109	+			TNF-α promoter	587 IBD, 304 UC, 241 CD/NOD2–	–857C associated with IBD and UC by TDT, and with IBD, UC and CD/NOD2– by case-control	UK
110	+			TNF-α (–308 G/A, –238 G/A)	124 CD, 106 UC, 111 controls	Haplotype AG (–308A/–238G) in UC ($P < 0.01$)	Japanese
111			7p21	IL-6 (–174 G/C)	169 CD, 133 UC, 440 controls	No IBD associations	German
113	+		10q11.21	MBL (mutations in exon 1)	287 CD, 142 UC, 308 controls	Frequency of mutations lower in UC vs. CD ($P = 0.01$) or controls ($P = 0.02$)	Belgian
112		IBD2	12q13	β7 integrin (4 SNPs tested)	300 CD, 254 UC	No IBD association by TDT	UK
114			12q13–q14	Advillin (AVIL)	24 IBD patients with linkage evidence to IBD2	No IBD associated coding or flanking intron polymorphisms identified	German
115		IBD1	16p11–p12	CD11A-D (α-integrins)	369 IBD trios, 380 controls	A few weak associations in case-controls not found by TDT, 21 SNPs tested	German
58			16p12	IL-4RA (Q576R)	Sibpairs (16 CD, 71 UC, 37 mixed)	RR homozygotes decreased in UC and IBD vs. controls ($P = 0.038$)	Finnish

Ref.	Association	Locus	Chromosome	Gene/polymorphism	Samples tested	Findings	Ethnicity
91		IBD1	16p12	IL-4RA (Q576R)	221 CD, 147 UC, 446 controls	No IBD association (see IL-4, Klein)	German
92	+/–				86 CD, 98 UC, 321 controls	Association limited to combination with IL-4 −34T ($P = 0.005$) (see IL-4, Aithal)	UK
116	+	IBD6	19p13	ICAM-1 (R241G, K469E)	96 CD, 121 UC, 116 controls	R241 allele and UC ($P = 0.024$); EE homozygotes and CD ($P = 0.002$) and UC ($P = 0.037$)	German
117	+				79 CD, 128 UC, 103 controls	K469 allele frequency ($Pc = 0.0026$) and carriage ($Pc = 0.0034$) increased in IBD	Japanese
118			19q13	TGFB1	99 CD, 42 UC, 88 controls	No IBD associations or subphenotype associations	German
119	+		19q13.4	IL-11 promoter, allele 1	222 CD, 152 UC, 400 controls	Allele 1 of promoter repeat polymorphism associated with UC ($P < 0.002$)	German

Table 4. Recent non-human leukocyte antigen (HLA) candidate gene reports. *Pc*: corrected P-value. No IBD associations: no inflammatory bowel disease (IBD), Crohn's disease (CD), or ulcerative colitis (UC) associations; NOD2–: persons without NOD2 mutations. APC: adenomatous polyposis of the colon; AVIL: advillin; CCR: CC chemokine receptor; CTLA: cytotoxic T lymphocyte-associated; ICAM: intracellular adhesion molecule; IL: interleukin; MBL: mannose-binding lectin; MICA: MHC class I chain-related gene A; MICB: MHC class I chain-related gene B; MLH: MutL homolog; NRAMP: natural resistance-associated macrophage protein; SNP: single nucleotide polymorphism; TDT: transmission/disequilibrium test; TNF: tumor necrosis factor.

spanned these two loci, Dechairo et al. [51] re-genotyped an extended familial IBD cohort that included the original 1996, Oxford University genome-screen pedigrees [44].

In this report [51], evidence for both the 3p and 7q loci was decreased in comparison with the initial genome screen study (MLS chromosome 3p, 1.25 vs. 2.69; MLS chromosome 7q, 1.26 vs. 3.08). The additional information provided by use of the high-density marker set also decreased linkage evidence within the original genome-screen subset of patients.

Four other studies have found replication evidence for linkage within or proximal to the original chromosome 3p locus region identified in the first Oxford University genome-wide screen (see **Table 2**) [44]. In two studies, there was evidence for replication near the more centromeric region of the original 3p locus. In the Canadian genome-wide screen there was suggestive evidence of linkage (MLS 2.4) at 3p21, 10 cM centromeric to the original Oxford University locus [50]. In a Finnish population study, Paavola et al. performed linkage analyses to determine if there was evidence for previously identified putative IBD loci on chromosomes 1p, 3p, 3q, 7, 12 (IBD2), 14 (IBD4), and 16 (IBD1). Besides being from a relatively isolated population, their cohort was unique in that the majority of multiplex pedigrees were UC as opposed to CD. There was evidence to support linkage to the chromosome 3p locus at 3p21; maximum linkage evidence was observed at D3S2432 (MLS 1.68, $P = 0.0027$) [58]. There was also nominal evidence for linkage on chromosomes 3q (D3S2427, $P = 0.031$), 16p (CD-only pedigrees, D16S407, $P = 0.019$), and 1p (IBD7, D1S552, $P = 0.021$). The 1p and 3q loci overlapped those identified in our IBD genome screen [55]. Interestingly, the 1p/IBD7 linkage evidence in this Finnish population was most pronounced using a dominant model.

More recently, using the same German/UK IBD pedigrees as used in their fine-mapping study of the 6p locus [49], Hampe et al. genotyped chromosome 3p at high density and found evidence for linkage replication at D3S1283 (MLS 1.40) [60], within the Oxford University 3p interval, but more centromeric. Even greater linkage evidence was observed in CD families at marker D3S1304 (3p25) (MLS 1.65), just p-telomeric to the original Oxford University 3p locus interval [44] – and on the opposite side of the locus as the Canadian and Finnish 3p replications [50].

Finally, a recent University of Pittsburgh collaborative North American study [59] found evidence for a CD locus at 3p26, 10 cM p-telomeric to the 3p25 finding in the Hampe et al. 3p locus replication study [60]. The Pittsburgh group reanalyzed their previously reported 5 cM genome-wide screen of 127 CD affected sibling pairs [54] for evidence of increased transmission of specific microsatellite alleles to sibling-pair offspring by use of TDT (using the program TDTLIKE) [59]. They identified one marker with significant distorted transmission of alleles (D3S1297) at a genome-wide corrected $P = 0.039$ (nominal $P = 0.000052$). They then added additional pedigrees to a larger set of 234 IBD pedigrees containing 190 CD-only families, 29 UC-only families, and 53 mixed families. They genotyped these families using 16 closely spaced microsatellite markers. They observed strong evidence of linkage (MLS 3.78). Evidence was contributed by all IBD phenotypes. There were also significant transmission/ disequilibrium results at two adjacent markers (D3S3525 and a novel microsatellite marker).

In summary, these multiple studies show chromosome 3p linkage evidence [44,50,51,58–60] and suggest that there may be two chromosome 3p IBD loci: a locus at 3p25–3p26 and a locus more centromeric at 3p21.

X-chromosome linkage

CD is more frequent in females than males (ratio 1.3:1), and IBD is more frequent in patients with Turner's syndrome (an X-linked syndrome). Only one genome-wide screen has found any linkage evidence on chromosome X: the German/UK screen reported nominal evidence for linkage at Xp21 and Xq25 (MLS 1.59 and 1.71, respectively) [56]. However, several of the other genome-wide screens either did not genotype or did not analyze the X chromosome for linkage.

Vermeire et al. screened 79 Belgian pedigrees (68 CD, 11 mixed) specifically for chromosome X, and found evidence for linkage in the pericentromeric region (MLS 2.5, $P = 0.0003$) [120]. The remainder of the X chromosome was excluded (LOD exclusion –2). Additional markers were then used to refine linkage, which was maximum at DXS1203 ($P = 0.0017$).

These results did not overlap with the German/UK findings – though the latter depended on linkage evidence from UC pedigrees. Further investigations are needed to determine the significance of these initial chromosome X findings.

HLA genes

Table 1 summarizes replicated or strongly positive HLA association studies. Common patterns of association are beginning to emerge. UC has been associated with HLA-DR2 serotypes [22–25] and genotypes (DRB1*15 [19], DRB1*1501 [26], and DRB1*1502 [9,11,27,28]) in multiple populations (including European, Ashkenazim, and Japanese), with particularly consistent associations in the Japanese population [11,22–24,27].

HLA-DR1 genotype, DRB1*0103, has been associated with UC in multiple Caucasian populations [9,10,18–20] and was also associated with CD in three studies [8–10]. Recently, Silverberg et al. observed that the strong DRB1*0103 association with CD observed in non-Jewish Canadian patients (odds ratio [OR] 5.23, $P = 0.0007$) was primarily from those patients with CD limited to the colon (DRB1*0103 allele in colon-only CD patients, 35.7%; in ileal-involvement CD patients, 9.7%; colon-only OR 5.2, $P = 0.02$) [10]. Thus, DRB1*0103 may be a risk factor for IBD (CD or UC) limited to the colon. The same is not true for HLA-DR2, which appears to be UC specific. In fact, in recent studies, DRB1*1501 was found to be inversely associated with CD [11,12]. For CD, the three most consistent associations have been with HLA-DRB1*07 [8,12,15,16], HLA-DRB1*1302 [14,17], and HLA-DRB1*03 (an inverse association) [8,15–17].

A meta-analysis on both HLA serotypes and genotypes by Stokkers et al. confirmed these general observations [121]. UC was most strongly associated with DR2 (OR 2.00) – and specifically for genotype DRB1*1502 (OR 3.74) – and with DR1 genotype DRB1*0103 (OR 3.42), DR9 (OR 1.54), and DR4 (OR 0.54; an inverse association). CD associations were noted for DRB3*0301 (OR 2.18), DR7 (OR 1.42), and DQ4 (OR 1.88), and inverse associations with DR3 (OR 0.71) and DR2 (OR 0.83).

HLA genetic polymorphisms and phenotypic expression

Many studies have evaluated variations in phenotypic expression (ie, site, disease behavior, and extraintestinal disease) and HLA genetic polymorphisms. These observations are most significant when the HLA polymorphism is found to also have an overall association with IBD, UC, or CD. Some polymorphisms (eg, HLA-B27) may not increase risk for IBD, but rather result in increased risk for specific IBD-related disease manifestations, such as spondyloarthropathy.

Several reports have observed an association between DRB1*0103 and extensive UC, severe UC requiring colectomy, and type I peripheral arthropathy (ie, self-limited large joint acute inflammatory arthritis) [19,20]. In the same UK population, Orchard et al. found that in addition to DRB1*0301 (relative risk [RR] 12.1), HLA-B27 (RR 4.0) and HLA-B*35 (RR 2.2) were also associated with type I arthropathy [122]. Type II peripheral arthritis (chronic arthritis involving five or more joints) was associated with HLA-B44 (RR 2.1). In a further evaluation of extraintestinal IBD, patients with IBD and a history of ocular inflammatory episodes (iritis, episcleritis, or uveitis) were more likely to carry HLA-B27 (RR 4.5), HLA-DRB1*0103 (RR 3.2), or HLA-B58 (RR 13.1) [123]. Erythema nodosum was significantly associated only with the TNF-α promoter polymorphism −1031C. TNF-α promoter polymorphisms were not associated with ocular inflammation.

In this same population, Ahmad et al. reported an association of DRB1*0701 and ileal disease (RR 1.61, P = 0.02) [12]. This association was particularly strong in patients without *NOD2* mutations (DRB1*0701/*NOD2*-negative risk of ileal disease was RR 2.2, P = 0.0009). Bouma et al. reported that the inverse association between CD and HLA-DRB1*03 (as observed in several studies) was specifically strong for protection against developing perianal CD (OR 0.09, P = 0.005) [29].

TNF-α and MHC class I chain-related gene A

In addition to the HLA genes, several groups have made progress in studying two other genes in the HLA 6p21 IBD3 region: TNF-α and MHC class I chain-related gene A (MICA) (see **Table 4**).

TNF-α

TNF-α is located between HLA-B and HLA-DR, and is a potent mediator of inflammation. In IBD, TNF-α plays a crucial role as a proinflammatory cytokine. The efficacy of monoclonal anti-TNF-α antibody in treating CD has spurred interest in potential influences of TNF genetic variations.

Initial research using regional microsatellites found evidence for an association of TNF with CD [124]. More recently, interest has shifted to genetic analysis of specific functional promoter variants that appear to regulate TNF-α gene expression, particularly −308 G/A and −857 C/T. A recent population study in Japanese patients found an association of a TNF-α promoter haplotype (−308A/−238G) and TNF receptor superfamily member 1B gene variants (TNFR2) (1466 A/G, 1493 C/T) with UC and CD, respectively (P < 0.01, P < 0.05) (see **Table 4**) [110]. This contrasts with a previous population study in Dutch patients that demonstrated a lower frequency of –308A polymorphism in UC patients as compared with controls [125].

TNF-α promoter –857

A positive association of TNF-α promoter –857C with CD was initially reported in a small Japanese case-control study [126], but a significant effect of this allele was not observed with a larger Japanese cohort (154 CD, 265 controls) [127].

In northern European Caucasian families, a genetic association of TNF –857C promoter polymorphism with IBD was recently reported [109]. IBD was associated with this promoter variant in 556 IBD trios by TDT ($P = 0.004$); these results were replicated in a separate cohort of 130 IBD patients and 278 controls ($P = 0.029$). Additionally, TNF –857C was associated with both UC and CD in case-control analyses for the total set of 304 UC cases ($P = 0.001$) and 241 CD cases ($P = 0.0022$), but only in those CD patients without *NOD2* mutations. The authors also showed increased whole-blood TNF production in healthy TNF –857C homozygotes, and that transcription factor OCT1 (octamer-binding transcription factor 1) bound TNF –857T-containing but not TNF –857C-containing oligonucleotides.

Considering the difference in CD phenotype between Japanese and Caucasian populations, and the rarity of *NOD2* variants in Japanese CD patients [77,78], the genetic mechanism of inheritance for TNF might differ in these two populations. It must also be remembered that, due to strong linkage disequilibrium throughout the HLA region, intensive genetic analysis will be needed to determine if the observed TNF-α associations are not causal, but secondary to associations with variants of other nearby genes in linkage disequilibrium.

MICA

MICA is located close to HLA-B. Groh et al. found that MICA and the closely related gene B (MICB) regulate protective responses of γ/δ T cells in the epithelium of the intestinal tract [128]. In a Japanese UC population, an association was observed between the A6 form of a MICA transmembrane triplet repeat and disease susceptibility, particularly in early-onset disease (P value corrected for multiple alleles tested [Pc] = 0.0042) [108].

Orchard et al. investigated the microsatellite polymorphism MICA allele 7 (MICA*007) in 50 UC and 50 CD patients [129]. MICA*007 was present at significantly higher frequency in the UC patients (Pc = 0.003) than controls. Note that MICA*007 is in linkage disequilibrium with HLA-B*27. However, in a larger and more comprehensive study, these results could not be extended: Ahmad et al. reported an analysis of 48 MICA and 17 MICB alleles in 248 CD patients, 329 UC patients, and 354 controls [107]. No significant associations were observed.

IL-1 receptor antagonist

The IL-1 gene family on chromosome 2q14 encodes IL-1α (*IL1A*), IL-1β (*IL1B*), and the IL-1 receptor antagonist (*IL1RN*). IL-1 regulates activation of the mucosal immune system and the production of inflammatory cytokines.

Several studies have found a significant association of UC with allele 2 of an 86-bp tandem repeat segment of the *IL1RN* gene (IL1RN*2); however, a significant number of studies have not [94]. Variability in results might arise from different sample sizes or patients with different ethnic backgrounds.

Carter et al. performed a meta-analysis of seven previously reported studies in northern Europeans, and a new set of 320 UC patients and 827 controls from the UK [94]. For the total meta-analysis set – which included 910 UC patients and 1925 controls – there was a significant IL1RN*2/UC association (OR 1.23, P = 0.01), though the genetic effect was weak.

In a follow-up study by the same group, there was a stronger association between IL1RN*2 and risk for pouchitis observed among 82 UC patients followed prospectively for pouchitis following ileal pouch–anal anastomosis [130]. By the Cox proportional hazard model, relative hazard was 3.1 ($P = 0.02$).

A further study, which was not included in the meta-analysis, examined 529 northern European Caucasian patients with IBD (347 UC, 182 CD) and 289 racially and geographically matched healthy controls. This study found slightly lower allele 2 rates in the UC patients [95]. Additionally, a recent Belgian population study (124 UC, 218 CD, and 401 controls) also showed no association with allele 2, but rather found a significant decrease in the frequency of allele 1 ($P = 0.048$) in UC patients as compared with controls [96]. Thus, the association observed in the meta-analysis of Carter et al. may be related to publication bias.

Overall, it must be considered that if there is a UC and IL1RN*2 association, then it is very weak. The association may be with a specific subphenotype of UC, such as pouchitis, it may require the presence of other genetic or specific environmental cofactors, or it may be related to an overall process of inflammation associated with UC as well as other inflammatory disease. For example, a recent study found an association of IL1RN*2 in 106 Dutch ankylosing spondylitis patients as compared with 104 healthy controls (OR 1.60, $P = 0.031$) [131]. Finally, a more rigorous within-family control study with TDT analysis may help to clarify the variations in IL1RN*2–UC association results.

CC chemokine receptor 5

There has been great interest in the CC chemokine receptor (CCR)5 gene located on chromosome 3p21.3, especially as linkage has been reported in the area, as noted above. CCR5 promotes specific leukocyte recruitment to the tissue during chronic inflammation, and recent studies revealed the association of a 32-bp deletion in the *CCR5* gene (CCR5-Δ32) with nonsevere rheumatoid arthritis and protection from HIV-1 [132,133]. However, as noted in **Table 4**, multiple studies have observed no associations (positive or negative) with this allele and IBD, CD, or UC. It is unlikely that further investigation of this allele is warranted, save for variations in subphenotypes such as severity, extent, and disease behavior.

Intercellular adhesion molecule-1

ICAM-1 maps to the chromosome 19p13, IBD6 region. The protein is expressed on vascular endothelium and plays a key role in transendothelial migration of neutrophils.

A report by Yang et al. found no overall association of the ICAM-1-coding polymorphism R241G (found within a key functional domain) with either UC or CD [134]. However, the R241 allele was found more frequently in pANCA-negative UC and pANCA-positive CD – a seemingly inconsistent association.

ICAM-1 was re-examined in a German population study [116], in which the R241 allele was found to be associated with UC. Patients homozygous (EE) at another polymorphic site, K469E, were at greater risk for both CD and UC (P = 0.002 and P = 0.037, respectively). Associations were independent of pANCA status.

Most recently, Matsuzawa et al. investigated both the R241G and K469E polymorphisms in a Japanese IBD population (79 CD, 128 UC, and 103 controls) [117]. Paradoxically, the K469 allele (as opposed to the E469 variant) was strongly associated with IBD patients as compared with controls (Pc = 0.0026). This increase was found in both CD and UC, particularly for extensive disease. The seemingly opposite German and Japanese ICAM-1 associations can be explained by: the presence of a noncoding ICAM-1 regulatory polymorphism or a polymorphism in a nearby gene in linkage disequilibrium with different alleles in the two different populations at amino acid 469; interactions of ICAM-1 with different genes in the two populations; or one or both results are false positive. Additional association studies, functional studies, and perhaps haplotype analyses may help to clarify these findings.

Interleukin-11

The anti-inflammatory cytokine IL-11 is a cytoprotective factor that down-regulates NF-κB. IL-11 also maps to chromosome 19. Klein et al. observed an association of UC with the 1 allele – $(GT)_7$ $(CT)_8$ – of a dinucleotide repeat promoter polymorphism (OR 1.21, $P < 0.002$) [119]. It is not known if this polymorphism is important to gene expression or regulation. A novel IL-11 coding polymorphism, R112H, was discovered. The H112 allele was in linkage disequilibrium with promoter allele 1; however, an observed increased presence of H112 in UC did not reach statistical significance [119].

Other candidate gene investigations

Table 4 notes four other candidate genes with positive IBD associations: human MutL homolog (MLH)1; natural resistance-associated macrophage protein (NRAMP)1; and mannose-binding lectin (MBL). *MLH1* is the DNA mismatch repair gene implicated in hereditary nonpolyposis colon cancer [135].

MLH1

In a relatively small study (45 CD patients, 36 UC patients, and 45 controls), Pokorny et al. studied two microsatellite polymorphisms and one exon polymorphism located near or within the *MLH1* gene [136]. They found that specific *MLH1* haplotypes of intragenic dinucleotide repeat marker D3S1611, MLH1 flanking marker D3S1768, and an exon 15 polymorphism were associated with the presence of CD and UC [136]. No adjustments were performed for the many haplotypes observed, and thus it is unclear if significance (strongest was $P = 0.002$ for a D3S1611 and exon 15 haplotype and CD vs. controls) would remain after adjustment for multiple testing. In a slightly larger study, Annese et al. recently reported genetic associations of the same *MLH1* microsatellites in Italian IBD patients [99]. Given the increased risk of IBD and colorectal cancer, these findings are provocative and will require more intensive investigation.

NRAMP1

NRAMP1 (located at chromosome 2q35) regulates metal ion transport and functions in controlling resistance to intracellular pathogens. The NRAMP2 isoform, which maps within the IBD2 locus, was previously found not to be associated with IBD [137]. A NRAMP1 gene promoter region encodes a Z-DNA forming, highly polymorphic, complex dinucleotide repeat [98].

Allele 2 of this promoter polymorphism has been associated with low NRAMP1 activity and susceptibility to rheumatoid arthritis and type 1 diabetes. Allele 3 has been associated with high activity and susceptibility to infectious diseases such as tuberculosis. Initial evidence from a Japanese study indicates that neither of these alleles were associated with IBD [98]. However, there was an association of the infrequent allele 7, function unknown, with both CD (allele frequency 11.1%, $Pc = 0.015$) and UC (allele frequency 11.2%, $P = 0.018$) as compared with controls (allele frequency 4.5%) [98]. Given the associations of NRAMP1 with other autoimmune diseases and infectious diseases, further investigations will be of interest.

MBL

MBL is located on the long arm of chromosome 10 (10q11.2–q21). MBL is thought to serve as a key factor in innate mucosal immune responses, and functions in recognizing a range of pathogens, including bacteria, yeasts, parasites, and some viruses.

Rector et al. investigated the distribution of MBL point mutations in codons 52, 54, and 57 of exon 1 in IBD patients and controls [113]. These mutations are associated with decreased MBL plasma concentrations and increased susceptibility to various infectious diseases. The frequency of the investigated MBL variants was significantly lower in UC patients as compared with CD patients

($P = 0.01$) and controls ($P = 0.02$). This suggests that functional MBL mutations may play a protective role against sporadic UC.

Others

The remaining recent candidate gene reports (**Table 4**) were all essentially negative studies. These reports included IL-10 [93], cytotoxic T lymphocyte-associated 4 (*CTLA4*) gene [97], the adenomatous polyposis of the colon (*APC*) gene [103], IL-6 [111], β7 integrin [112] and advillin (*AVIL*) [114] within the IBD2 locus, CD11 A–D α integrins [115] and IL-4 receptor [91] within the IBD1 locus, and transforming growth factor-β1 [118] within the IBD6 locus. All are IBD candidate genes with either demonstrated or suspected roles in IBD pathophysiology.

IL-10 is a key cytokine in suppressing inflammation. A UK study that demonstrated no association between IL-10 and IBD [93] was consistent with a previous German study [138]. However, given the importance of this gene in relation to IBD, a careful screen for functional variants is still required, followed by genetic testing in IBD.

CTLA4 also has inhibitory functions and codes for a cell surface molecule that down-regulates T-cell activation [97]. The A49G missense polymorphism has been associated with several autoimmune diseases, including celiac disease, both Hashimoto's thyroiditis and Graves' disease, and type 1 diabetes. Recently, this and a promoter polymorphism were found not to be associated with either Dutch UC or CD patients, nor with a small number (N = 40) of Chinese UC patients versus ethnically matched controls [97].

The β7 integrin lymphocyte homing gene represents an important IBD2, chromosome 12 candidate gene. The recent negative results from a thorough search for gene variants and association testing in a large set of within-family controls by Van Heel et al. [112] suggests that investigators will need to primarily focus on other IBD2 candidate genes, particularly those that map within more refined IBD2 linkage regions.

Another IBD2 candidate gene is *AVIL*, a member of the gelsolin/villin family of actin regulatory proteins, highly expressed in intestinal tissue. Tumer et al. sequenced the coding exons and flanking introns of the *AVIL* gene in patients from 24 IBD pedigrees with increased linkage evidence to IBD2 [114]. No disease-associated variants were identified. This initial study suggests that functional mutations in the coding region of AVIL are likely to be rare, although potential promoter, regulatory, and functional intronic polymorphisms cannot be excluded.

The essentially negative (when considering multiple testing) results of recent IL-4 receptor association studies [58,91,92] confirm the negative results of a larger previous study of multiple IL-4 receptor SNPs evaluated in 355 IBD families [139]. Additionally, the negative study of CD11 A–D by Frenzel et al. [115] (see **Table 4**), which was a large mutation investigation followed by both familial and case-control association analyses, suggests that other genes will require investigation if there is continued interest (as noted by Hampe et al. [86]) in the 16p11–12, p-centromeric region of the IBD1 locus.

Future directions in IBD genetics

IBD genetics is a very rapidly moving field. In the beginning months of 2003, there have already been several new studies, including further replication of the IBD5 haplotype [140], identification of potential new *NOD2* risk polymorphisms [141] and muramyl dipeptide as the bacterial cell wall component responsible for *NOD2* activation [142], and even more candidate gene studies [143,144]. These and other IBD genetic studies will be explored in detail in the next edition of the *IBD Yearbook*.

What exciting discoveries are likely to develop in IBD genetics over the next few years? Large, collaborative genome screens, utilizing over 1,000 IBD pedigrees and analyzing for subphenotypes of IBD (eg, ileal disease site or fistulizing disease behavior) or gene–gene interactions (ie, stratified by *NOD2* status) are planned.

Investigators will soon utilize new technologies, particularly high-density SNP genome screens. IBD genome screens with thousands of SNPs (<1 cM mapping density) could simultaneously test for both linkage and genome-wide association by TDT analyses.

Many previously overlooked genes, some in linkage areas, will likely be targeted for candidate gene study as investigators perform large-scale functional analyses and identify additional genes that are altered in IBD. For example, recent cDNA microarray studies have found multiple genes differentially expressed in IBD, CD, and UC phenotypes [145,146]. New microarray studies will include many uncharacterized genes (such as those known only as expressed sequence tags) and may also detail how expression differences are associated with specific IBD pathophysiological mechanisms. Results from these studies may suggest more specific genetic analyses, perhaps looking for epistatic interactions with other genes shown to biologically interact with the novel gene of interest.

Finally, as our understanding of the specific risks of IBD susceptibility gene variants becomes established, we will likely see changes in the clinical arena with diagnosis, prediction of disease course, medical therapies, and potentially preventive treatments all implemented on the basis of individual patient IBD susceptibility gene profiles.

References

1. Crohn BB. Broadening concept of regional enteritis. *Am J Dig Dis* 1934;1:97–9.
2. Mayberry JF, Rhodes J, Newcombe RG. Familial prevalence of inflammatory bowel disease in relatives of patients with Crohn's disease. *BMJ* 1980;280:84.
3. Orholm M, Munkholm P, Langholz E et al. Familial occurrence of inflammatory bowel disease. *N Engl J Med* 1991;324:84–8.
4. Mertz HR, Peterson WL, Walsh JH. "Familial hyperpepsinogenemia" and *Helicobacter pylori* infection. *Am J Gastroenterol* 2000;95:943–6.
5. Tysk C, Lindberg E, Jarnerot G et al. Ulcerative colitis and Crohn's disease in an unselected population of monozygotic and dizygotic twins. A study of heritability and the influence of smoking. *Gut* 1988;29:990–6.
6. Ahmad T, Satsangi J, McGovern D et al. Review article: the genetics of inflammatory bowel disease. *Aliment Pharmacol Ther* 2001;15:731–48.

7. Breslin NP, Todd A, Kilgallen C et al. Monozygotic twins with Crohn's disease and ulcerative colitis: a unique case report. *Gut* 1997;41:557–60.

8. Danze PM, Colombel JF, Jacquot S et al. Association of HLA class II genes with susceptibility to Crohn's disease. *Gut* 1996;39:69–72.

9. Trachtenberg EA, Yang H, Hayes E et al. HLA class II haplotype associations with inflammatory bowel disease in Jewish (Ashkenazi) and non-Jewish caucasian populations. *Hum Immunol* 2000;61:326–33.

10. Silverberg MS, Mirea L, Bull SB et al. A population- and family-based study of Canadian families reveals association of HLA DRB1*0103 with colonic involvement in inflammatory bowel disease. *Inflamm Bowel Dis* 2003;9:1–9.

11. Yoshitake S, Kimura A, Okada M et al. HLA class II alleles in Japanese patients with inflammatory bowel disease. *Tissue Antigens* 1999;53:350–8.

12. Ahmad T, Armuzzi A, Bunce M et al. The molecular classification of the clinical manifestations of Crohn's disease. *Gastroenterology* 2002;122:854–66.

13. Nakajima A, Matsuhashi N, Kodama T et al. HLA-linked susceptibility and resistance genes in Crohn's disedase. *Gastroenterology* 1995;109:1462–7.

14. Forcione DG, Sands B, Isselbacher KJ et al. An increased risk of Crohn's disease in individuals who inherit the HLA class II DRB3*0301 allele. *Proc Natl Acad Sci USA* 1996;93:5094–8.

15. Reinshagen M, Loelliger C, Kuhn R et al. HLA class II gene frequencies in Crohn's disease: a population based analysis in Germany. *Gut* 1996;38:538–42.

16. Lombardi ML, Pirozzi G, Luongo V et al. Crohn disease: susceptibility and disease heterogeneity revealed by HLA genotyping. *Hum Immunol* 2001;62:701–4.

17. Gulwani-Akolkar B, Akolkar PN, Lin XY et al. HLA class II alleles associated with susceptibility and resistance to Crohn's disease in the Jewish population. *Inflamm Bowel Dis* 2000;6:71–6.

18. Satsangi J, Welsh KI, Bunce M et al. Contribution of genes of the major histocompatibility complex to susceptibility and disease phenotype in inflammatory bowel disease. *Lancet* 1996;347:1212–7.

19. Bouma G, Crusius JB, Garcia-Gonzalez MA et al. Genetic markers in clinically well defined patients with ulcerative colitis (UC). *Clin Exp Immunol* 1999;115:294–300.

20. Roussomoustakaki M, Satsangi J, Welsh K et al. Genetic markers may predict disease behavior in patients with ulcerative colitis. *Gastroenterology* 1997;112:1845–53.

21. Yamamoto-Furusho JK, Uscanga LF, Vargas-Alarcon G et al. Clinical and genetic heterogeneity in Mexican patients with ulcerative colitis. *Hum Immunol* 2003;64:119–23.

22. Asakura H, Tsuchiya M, Aiso S et al. Association of the human lymphocyte-DR2 antigen with Japanese ulcerative colitis. *Gastroenterology* 1982;82:413–8.

23. Kobayashi K, Atoh M, Konoeda Y et al. HLA-DR, DQ and T cell antigen receptor constant beta genes in Japanese patients with ulcerative colitis. *Clin Exp Immunol* 1990;80:400–3.

24. Toyoda H, Wang SJ, Yang HY et al. Distinct associations of HLA class II genes with inflammatory bowel disease. *Gastroenterology* 1993;104:741–8.

25. Yang H, Rotter JI, Toyoda H et al. Ulcerative colitis: a genetically heterogeneous disorder defined by genetic (HLA class II) and subclinical (antineutrophil cytoplasmic antibodies) markers. *J Clin Invest* 1993;92:1080–84.

26. Hirv K, Seyfarth M, Uibo R et al. Polymorphisms in tumour necrosis factor and adhesion molecule genes in patients with inflammatory bowel disease: associations with HLA-DR and -DQ alleles and subclinical markers. *Scand J Gastroenterol* 1999;34:1025–32.

27. Futami S, Aoyama N, Honsako Y et al. HLA-DRB1*1502 allele, subtype of DR15, is associated with susceptibility to ulcerative colitis and its progression. *Dig Dis Sci* 1995;40:814–8.

28. Uyar FA, Imeryuz N, Saruhan-Direskeneli G et al. The distribution of HLA-DRB alleles in ulcerative colitis patients in Turkey. *Eur J Immunogenet* 1998;25:293–6.

29. Bouma G, Poen AC, Garcia-Gonzalez MA et al. HLA-DRB1*03, but not the TNFA -308 promoter gene polymorphism, confers protection against fistulising Crohn's disease. *Immunogenetics* 1998;47:451–5.

30. Cho JH, Brant SR. Genetics and Genetic Markers in IBD. *Curr Opin Gastroenterol* 1998;14:283–88.

31. Yang H, Rotter JI. Genetics of inflammatory bowel disease. In: Targan SR, Shanahan F, editors. *Inflammatory Bowel Disease: from Bench to Bedside*. Baltimore, MD: Williams & Wilkins, 1994:32–64.

32. Karban A, Eliakim R, Brant SR. Genetics of inflammatory bowel disease. *Isr Med Assoc J* 2002;4:798–802.

33. Lander E, Kruglyak L. Genetic dissection of complex traits: guidelines for interpreting and reporting linkage results. *Nat Genet* 1995;11:241–7.

34. Hugot JP, Laurent-Puig P, Gower-Rousseau C et al. Mapping of a susceptibility locus for Crohn's disease on chromosome 16. *Nature* 1996;379:821–3.

35. Ohmen JD, Yang HY, Yamamoto KK et al. Susceptibility locus for inflammatory bowel disease on chromosome 16 has a role in Crohn's disease, but not in ulcerative colitis. *Hum Mol Genet* 1996;5:1679–83.

36. Parkes M, Satsangi J, Lathrop GM et al. Susceptibility loci in inflammatory bowel disease. *Lancet* 1996;348:1588.

37. Brant SR, Fu Y, Fields CT et al. American families with Crohn's disease have strong evidence for linkage to chromosome 16 but not chromosome 12. *Gastroenterology* 1998;115:1056–61.

38. Curran ME, Lau KF, Hampe J et al. Genetic analysis of inflammatory bowel disease in a large European cohort supports linkage to chromosomes 12 and 16. *Gastroenterology* 1998;115:1066–71.

39. Cavanaugh JA, Callen DF, Wilson SR et al. Analysis of Australian Crohn's disease pedigrees refines the localization for susceptibility to inflammatory bowel disease on chromosome 16. *Ann Hum Genet* 1998;62:291–8.

40. Annese V, Latiano A, Bovio P et al. Genetic analysis in Italian families with inflammatory bowel disease supports linkage to the IBD1 locus – a GISC study. *Eur J Hum Genet* 1999;7:567–73.

41. Brant SR, Panhuysen CI, Bailey-Wilson JE et al. Linkage heterogeneity for the IBD1 locus in Crohn's disease pedigrees by disease onset and severity. *Gastroenterology* 2000;119:1483–90.

42. Akolkar PN, Gulwani-Akolkar B, Lin XY et al. The IBD1 locus for susceptibility to Crohn's disease has a greater impact in Ashkenazi Jews with early onset disease *Am J Gastroenterol* 2001;96:1127–32.

43. Cavanaugh J. International collaboration provides convincing linkage replication in complex disease through analysis of a large pooled data set: Crohn disease and chromosome 16. *Am J Hum Genet* 2001;68:1165–71.

44. Satsangi J, Parkes M, Louis E et al. Two stage genome-wide search in inflammatory bowel disease provides evidence for susceptibility loci on chromosomes 3, 7 and 12. *Nat Genet* 1996;14:199–202.

45. Duerr RH, Barmada MM, Zhang L et al. Linkage and association between inflammatory bowel disease and a locus on chromosome 12. *Am J Hum Genet* 1998;63:95–100.

46. Yang H, Ohmen JD, Ma Y et al. Additional evidence of linkage between Crohn's disease and a putative locus on chromosome 12. *Genet Med* 1999;1:194–8.

47. Parkes M, Barmada MM, Satsangi J et al. The IBD2 locus shows linkage heterogeneity between ulcerative colitis and Crohn disease. *Am J Hum Genet* 2000;67:1605–10.

48. Yang H, Plevy SE, Taylor K et al. Linkage of Crohn's disease to the major histocompatibility complex region is detected by multiple non-parametric analyses. *Gut* 1999;44:519–26.

49. Hampe J, Shaw SH, Saiz R et al. Linkage of inflammatory bowel disease to human chromosome 6p. *Am J Hum Genet* 1999;65:1647–55.

50. Rioux JD, Silverberg MS, Daly MJ et al. Genomewide search in Canadian families with inflammatory bowel disease reveals two novel susceptibility loci. *Am J Hum Genet* 2000;66:1863–70.

51. Dechairo B, Dimon C, van Heel D et al. Replication and extension studies of inflammatory bowel disease susceptibility regions confirm linkage to chromosome 6p (IBD3). *Eur J Hum Genet* 2001;9:627–33.

52. Fisher SA, Hampe J, MacPherson AJ et al. Sex stratification of an inflammatory bowel disease genome search shows male-specific linkage to the HLA region of chromosome 6. *Eur J Hum Genet* 2002;10:259–65.

53. Ma Y, Ohmen JD, Li Z et al. A genome-wide search identifies potential new susceptibility loci for Crohn's disease. *Inflamm Bowel Dis* 1999;5:271–8.

54. Duerr RH, Barmada MM, Zhang L et al. High-density genome scan in Crohn disease shows confirmed linkage to chromosome 14q11–12. *Am J Hum Genet* 2000;66:1857–62.

55. Cho JH, Nicolae DL, Gold LH et al. Identification of novel susceptibility loci for inflammatory bowel disease on chromosomes 1p, 3q, and 4q: evidence for epistasis between 1p and IBD1. *Proc Natl Acad Sci USA* 1998;95:7502–7.

56. Hampe J, Schreiber S, Shaw SH et al. A genomewide analysis provides evidence for novel linkages in inflammatory bowel disease in a large European cohort. *Am J Hum Genet* 1999;64:808–16.

57. Cho JH, Nicolae DL, Ramos R et al. Linkage and linkage disequilibrium in chromosome band 1p36 in American Chaldeans with inflammatory bowel disease. *Hum Mol Genet* 2000;9:1425–32.

58. Paavola P, Helio T, Kiuru M et al. Genetic analysis in Finnish families with inflammatory bowel disease supports linkage to chromosome 3p21. *Eur J Hum Genet* 2001;9:328–34.

59. Duerr RH, Barmada MM, Zhang L et al. Evidence for an inflammatory bowel disease locus on chromosome 3p26: linkage, transmission/disequilibrium, and partitioning of linkage. *Hum Mol Genet* 2002;11:2599–606.

60. Hampe J, Lynch NJ, Daniels S et al. Fine mapping of the chromosome 3p susceptibility locus in inflammatory bowel disease. *Gut* 2001;48:191–7.

61. Schulze TG, McMahon FJ. Genetic association mapping at the crossroads: which test and why? Overview and practical guidelines. *Am J Med Genet* 2002;114:1–11.

62. Hugot JP, Chamaillard M, Zouali H et al. Association of NOD2 leucine-rich repeat variants with susceptibility to Crohn's disease. *Nature* 2001;411:599–603.

63. Ogura Y, Inohara N, Benito A et al. Nod2, a Nod1/Apaf-1 family member that is restricted to monocytes and activates NF-κB. *J Biol Chem* 2001;276:4812–8.

64. Podolsky DK. Inflammatory bowel disease. *N Engl J Med* 2002;347:417–29.

65. Ogura Y, Bonen DK, Inohara N et al. A frameshift mutation in NOD2 associated with susceptibility to Crohn's disease. *Nature* 2001;411:603–6.

66. Kuster W, Pascoe L, Purrmann J et al. The genetics of Crohn disease: complex segregation analysis of a family study with 265 patients with Crohn disease and 5,387 relatives. *Am J Med Genet* 1989;32:105–8.

67. Lesage S, Zouali H, Cezard JP et al. CARD15/NOD2 mutational analysis and genotype-phenotype correlation in 612 patients with inflammatory bowel disease. *Am J Hum Genet* 2002;70:845–57.

68. Bonen DK, Ogura Y, Nicolae DL et al. Crohn's disease-associated NOD2 variants share a signaling defect in response to lipopolysaccharide and peptidoglycan. *Gastroenterology* 2003;124:140–6.

69. Schreiber S, Nikolaus S, Hampe J. Activation of nuclear factor κB inflammatory bowel disease. *Gut* 1998;42:477–84.

70. Erdman S, Fox JG, Dangler CA et al. Typhlocolitis in NF-κB-deficient mice. *J Immunol* 2001;166:1443–7.

71. Cuthbert AP, Fisher SA, Mirza MM et al. The contribution of NOD2 gene mutations to the risk and site of disease in inflammatory bowel disease. *Gastroenterology* 2002;122:867–74.

72. Hampe J, Grebe J, Nikolaus S et al. Association of NOD2 (CARD 15) genotype with clinical course of Crohn's disease: a cohort study. *Lancet* 2002;359:1661–5.

73. Vermeire S, Wild G, Kocher K et al. CARD15 genetic variation in a Quebec population: prevalence, genotype-phenotype relationship, and haplotype structure. *Am J Hum Genet* 2002;71:74–83.

74. Abreu MT, Taylor KD, Lin YC et al. Mutations in NOD2 are associated with fibrostenosing disease in patients with Crohn's disease. *Gastroenterology* 2002;123:679–88.

75. Brant SR, Picco MF, Achkar JP et al. Crohn's Disease: Role of Nod2/Card15 gene mutations in clinical heterogeneity. *Am J Hum Genet* 2002;71:484.

76. Hampe J, Cuthbert A, Croucher PJ et al. Association between insertion mutation in NOD2 gene and Crohn's disease in German and British populations. *Lancet* 2001;357:1925–8.

77. Inoue N, Tamura K, Kinouchi Y et al. Lack of common NOD2 variants in Japanese patients with Crohn's disease. *Gastroenterology* 2002;123:86–91.

78. Yamazaki K, Takazoe M, Tanaka T et al. Absence of mutation in the NOD2/ CARD15 gene among 483 Japanese patients with Crohn's disease. *J Hum Genet* 2002;47:469–72.

79. Croucher PJ, Mascheretti S, Hampe J et al. Haplotype structure and association to Crohn's disease of CARD15 mutations in two ethnically divergent populations. *Eur J Hum Genet* 2003;11:6–16.

80. Sandler RS. Epidemiology. In: Targan SR, Shanahan F, editors. *Inflammatory Bowel Disease: from Bench to Bedside*. Baltimore: Williams & Wilkins, 1994:5–30.

81. Zhou Z, Lin XY, Akolkar PN et al. Variation at NOD2/CARD15 in familial and sporadic cases of Crohn's disease in the Ashkenazi Jewish population. *Am J Gastroenterol* 2002;97:3095–101.

82. Vermeire S, Louis E, Rutgeerts P et al. NOD2/CARD15 does not influence response to infliximab in Crohn's disease. *Gastroenterology* 2002;123:106–11.

83. Mascheretti S, Hampe J, Croucher PJ et al. Response to infliximab treatment in Crohn's disease is not associated with mutations in the CARD15 (NOD2) gene: an analysis in 534 patients from two multicenter, prospective GCP-level trials. *Pharmacogenetics* 2002;12:509–15.

84. Miceli-Richard C, Lesage S, Rybojad M et al. CARD15 mutations in Blau syndrome. *Nat Genet* 2001;29:19–20.

85. Wang X, Kuivaniemi H, Bonavita G et al. CARD15 mutations in familial granulomatosis syndromes: a study of the original Blau syndrome kindred and other families with large-vessel arteritis and cranial neuropathy. *Arthritis Rheum* 2002;46:3041–5.

86. Hampe J, Frenzel H, Mirza MM et al. Evidence for a NOD2-independent susceptibility locus for inflammatory bowel disease on chromosome 16p. *Proc Natl Acad Sci USA* 2002;99:321–6.

87. Williams CN, Kocher K, Lander ES et al. Using a genome-wide scan and meta-analysis to identify a novel IBD locus and confirm previously identified IBD loci. *Inflamm Bowel Dis* 2002;8:375–81.

88. Wise LH, Lanchbury JS, Lewis CM. Meta-analysis of genome searches. *Ann Hum Genet* 1999;63:263–72.

89. Lonjou C, Barnes K, Chen H et al. A first trial of retrospective collaboration for positional cloning in complex inheritance: assay of the cytokine region on chromosome 5 by the consortium on asthma genetics (COAG). *Proc Natl Acad Sci USA* 2000; 97:10942–7.

90. Rioux JD, Daly MJ, Silverberg MS et al. Genetic variation in the 5q31 cytokine gene cluster confers susceptibility to Crohn disease. *Nat Genet* 2001;29:223–8.

91. Klein W, Tromm A, Griga T et al. Interleukin-4 and interleukin-4 receptor gene polymorphisms in inflammatory bowel diseases. *Genes Immun* 2001;2:287–9.

92. Aithal GP, Day CP, Leathart J et al. Association of single nucleotide polymorphisms in the interleukin-4 gene and interleukin-4 receptor gene with Crohn's disease in a British population. *Genes Immun* 2001;2:44–7.

93. Aithal GP, Craggs A, Day CP et al. Role of polymorphisms in the interleukin-10 gene in determining disease susceptibility and phenotype in inflamatory bowel disease. *Dig Dis Sci* 2001;46:1520–5.

94. Carter MJ, di Giovine FS, Jones S et al. Association of the interleukin 1 receptor antagonist gene with ulcerative colitis in Northern European Caucasians. *Gut* 2001; 48:461–7.

95. Craggs A, West S, Curtis A et al. Absence of a genetic association between IL-1RN and IL-1B gene polymorphisms in ulcerative colitis and Crohn disease in multiple populations from northeast England. *Scand J Gastroenterol* 2001;36:1173–8.

96. Vijgen L, Van Gysel M, Rector A et al. Interleukin-1 receptor antagonist VNTR-polymorphism in inflammatory bowel disease. *Genes Immun* 2002;3:400–6.

97. Xia B, Crusius JB, Wu J et al. CTLA4 gene polymorphisms in Dutch and Chinese patients with inflammatory bowel disease. *Scand J Gastroenterol* 2002;37:1296–300.

98. Kojima Y, Kinouchi Y, Takahashi S et al. Inflammatory bowel disease is associated with a novel promoter polymorphism of natural resistance-associated macrophage protein 1 (NRAMP1) gene. *Tissue Antigens* 2001;58:379–84.

99. Annese V, Piepoli A, Andriulli A et al. Association of Crohn's disease and ulcerative colitis with haplotypes of the MLH1 gene in Italian inflammatory bowel disease patients. *J Med Genet* 2002;39:332–4.

100. Rector A, Vermeire S, Thoelen I et al. Analysis of the CC chemokine receptor 5 (CCR5) delta-32 polymorphism in inflammatory bowel disease. *Hum Genet* 2001;108:190–3.

101. Herfarth H, Pollok-Kopp B, Goke M et al. Polymorphism of CC chemokine receptors CCR2 and CCR5 in Crohn's disease. *Immunol Lett* 2001;77:113–7.

102. Craggs A, Welfare M, Donaldson PT et al. The CC chemokine receptor 5 delta32 mutation is not associated with inflammatory bowel disease (IBD) in NE England. *Genes Immun* 2001;2:114–6.

103. Silverberg MS, Clelland C, Murphy JE et al. Carrier rate of APC I1307K is not increased in inflammatory bowel disease patients of Ashkenazi Jewish origin. *Hum Genet* 2001; 108:205–10.

104. Obana N, Takahashi S, Kinouchi Y et al. Ulcerative colitis is associated with a promoter polymorphism of lipopolysaccharide receptor gene, CD14. *Scand J Gastroenterol* 2002; 37:699–704.

105. Klein W, Tromm A, Griga T et al. A polymorphism in the CD14 gene is associated with Crohn disease. *Scand J Gastroenterol* 2002;37:189–91.

106. Glas J, Martin K, Brunnler G et al. MICA, MICB and C1_4_1 polymorphism in Crohn's disease and ulcerative colitis. *Tissue Antigens* 2001;58:243–9.

107. Ahmad T, Marshall SE, Mulcahy-Hawes K et al. High resolution MIC genotyping: Design and application to the investigation of inflammatory bowel disease susceptibility. *Tissue Antigens* 2002;60:164–79.

108. Sugimura K, Ota M, Matsuzawa J et al. A close relationship of triplet repeat polymorphism in MHC class I chain-related gene A (MICA) to the disease susceptibility and behavior in ulcerative colitis. *Tissue Antigens* 2001;57:9–14.

109. van Heel DA, Udalova IA, De Silva AP et al. Inflammatory bowel disease is associated with a TNF polymorphism that affects an interaction between the OCT1 and NFkB transcription factors. *Hum Mol Genet* 2002;11:1281–9.

110. Sashio H, Tamura K, Ito R et al. Polymorphisms of the TNF gene and the TNF receptor superfamily member 1B gene are associated with susceptibility to ulcerative colitis and Crohn's disease, respectively. *Immunogenetics* 2002;53:1020–7.

111. Klein W, Tromm A, Griga T et al. The polymorphism at position -174 of the IL-6 gene is not associated with inflammatory bowel disease. *Eur J Gastroenterol Hepatol* 2001;13:45–7.

112. Van Heel DA, Carey AH, Jewell DP. Identification of novel polymorphisms in the β7 integrin gene: family-based association studies in inflammatory bowel disease. *Genes Immun* 2001;2:455–60.

113. Rector A, Lemey P, Laffut W et al. Mannan-binding lectin (MBL) gene polymorphisms in ulcerative colitis and Crohn's disease. *Genes Immun* 2001;2:323–8.

114. Tumer Z, Croucher PJ, Jensen LR et al. Genomic structure, chromosome mapping and expression analysis of the human AVIL gene, and its exclusion as a candidate for locus for inflammatory bowel disease at 12q13–14 (IBD2). *Gene* 2002;288:179–85.

115. Frenzel H, Hampe J, Huse K et al. Mutation detection and physical mapping of the CD11 gene cluster in association with inflammatory bowel disease. *Immunogenetics* 2002;53:835–42.

116. Braun C, Zahn R, Martin K et al. Polymorphisms of the ICAM-1 gene are associated with inflammatory bowel disease, regardless of the p-ANCA status. *Clin Immunol* 2001;101:357–60.

117. Matsuzawa J, Sugimura K, Matsuda Y et al. Association between K469E allele of intercellular adhesion molecule 1 gene and inflammatory bowel disease in a Japanese population. *Gut* 2003;52:75–8.

118. Schulte CM, Goebell H, Roher HD et al. C-509T polymorphism in the TGFB1 gene promoter: impact on Crohn's disease susceptibility and clinical course? *Immunogenetics* 2001;53:178–82.

119. Klein W, Tromm A, Griga T et al. A polymorphism in the IL11 gene is associated with ulcerative colitis. *Genes Immun* 2002;3:494–6.

120. Vermeire S, Satsangi J, Peeters M et al. Evidence for inflammatory bowel disease of a susceptibility locus on the X chromosome. *Gastroenterology* 2001;120:834–40.

121. Stokkers PC, Reitsma PH, Tytgat GN et al. HLA-DR and -DQ phenotypes in inflammatory bowel disease: a meta-analysis. *Gut* 1999;45:395–401.

122. Orchard TR, Thiyagaraja S, Welsh KI et al. Clinical phenotype is related to HLA genotype in the peripheral arthropathies of inflammatory bowel disease. *Gastroenterology* 2000;118:274–8.

123. Orchard TR, Chua CN, Ahmad T et al. Uveitis and erythema nodosum in inflammatory bowel disease: clinical features and the role of HLA genes. *Gastroenterology* 2002;123:714–8.

124. Plevy SE, Targan SR, Yang H et al. Tumor necrosis factor microsatellites define a Crohn's disease-associated haplotype on chromosome 6. *Gastroenterology* 1996;110:1053–60.

125. Bouma G, Xia B, Crusius JB et al. Distribution of four polymorphisms in the tumour necrosis factor (TNF) genes in patients with inflammatory bowel disease (IBD). *Clin Exp Immunol* 1996;103:391–6.

126. Negoro K, Kinouchi Y, Hiwatashi N et al. Crohn's disease is associated with novel polymorphisms in the 5′-flanking region of the tumor necrosis factor gene. *Gastroenterology* 1999;117:1062–8.

127. Kawasaki A, Tsuchiya N, Hagiwara K et al. Independent contribution of HLA-DRB1 and TNF-α promoter polymorphisms to the susceptibility to Crohn's disease. *Genes Immun* 2000;1:351–7.

128. Groh V, Steinle A, Bauer S et al. Recognition of stress-induced MHC molecules by intestinal epithelial gammadelta T cells. *Science* 1998;279:1737–40.

129. Orchard TR, Dhar A, Simmons JD et al. MHC class I chain-like gene A (MICA) and its associations with inflammatory bowel disease and peripheral arthropathy. *Clin Exp Immunol* 2001;126:437–40.

130. Carter MJ, di Giovine FS, Cox A et al. The interleukin 1 receptor antagonist gene allele 2 as a predictor of pouchitis following colectomy and IPAA in ulcerative colitis. *Gastroenterology* 2001;121:805–11.

131. van der Paardt M, Crusius JB, Garcia-Gonzalez MA et al. Interleukin-1β and interleukin-1 receptor antagonist gene polymorphisms in ankylosing spondylitis. *Rheumatology* 2002;41:1419–23.

132. Zapico I, Coto E, Rodriguez A et al. CCR5 (chemokine receptor-5) DNA-polymorphism influences the severity of rheumatoid arthritis. *Genes Immun* 2000;1:288–89.

133. Sullivan AD, Wigginton J, Kirschner D. The coreceptor mutation CCR5Delta32 influences the dynamics of HIV epidemics and is selected for by HIV. *Proc Natl Acad Sci USA* 2001;98:10214–9.

134. Yang H, Vora DK, Targan SR et al. Intercellular adhesion molecule 1 gene associations with immunologic subsets of inflammatory bowel disease. *Gastroenterology* 1995; 109:440–8.

135. Papadopoulos N, Nicolaides NC, Wei YF et al. Mutation of a mutL homolog in hereditary colon cancer. *Science* 1994;263:1625–9.

136. Pokorny RM, Hofmeister A, Galandiuk S et al. Crohn's disease and ulcerative colitis are associated with the DNA repair gene MLH1. *Ann Surg* 1997;225:718–23.

137. Stokkers PC, Huibregtse K Jr, Leegwater AC et al. Analysis of a positional candidate gene for inflammatory bowel disease: NRAMP2. *Inflamm Bowel Dis* 2000;6:92–8.

138. Klein W, Tromm A, Griga T et al. The IL-10 gene is not involved in the predisposition to inflammatory bowel disease. *Electrophoresis* 2000;21:3578–82.

139. Olavesen MG, Hampe J, Mirza MM et al. Analysis of single-nucleotide polymorphisms in the interleukin-4 receptor gene for association with inflammatory bowel disease. *Immunogenetics* 2000;51:1–7.

140. Negoro K, McGovern DP, Kinouchi Y et al. Analysis of the IBD5 locus and potential gene–gene interactions in Crohn's disease. *Gut* 2003;52:541–6.

141. Sugimura K, Taylor KD, Lin YC et al. A novel NOD2/CARD15 haplotype conferring risk for Crohn disease in Ashkenazi Jews. *Am J Hum Genet* 2003;72:509–18.

142. Inohara N, Ogura Y, Fontalba A et al. Host recognition of bacterial muramyl dipeptide mediated through NOD2. *J Biol Chem* 2003;278:5509–12.

143. Louis E, Michel V, Hugot JP et al. Early development of stricturing or penetrating pattern in Crohn's disease is influenced by disease location, number of flares, and smoking but not by NOD2/CARD15 genotype. *Gut* 2003;52:552–7.

144. Schwab M, Schaeffeler E, Marx C et al. Association between the C3435T MDR1 gene polymorphism and susceptibility for ulcerative colitis. *Gastroenterology* 2003;124:26–33.

145. Lawrance IC, Fiocchi C, Chakravarti S. Ulcerative colitis and Crohn's disease: distinctive gene expression profiles and novel susceptibility candidate genes. *Hum Mol Genet* 2001;10:445–56.

146. Uthoff SM, Eichenberger MR, Lewis RK et al. Identification of candidate genes in ulcerative colitis and Crohn's disease using cDNA array technology. *Int J Oncol* 2001;19:803–10.

5

Current status and new imaging trends in IBD

Karl Turetschek & Christoph Gasche

Introduction

Imaging in inflammatory bowel disease (IBD) serves two major purposes: first, to establish the primary diagnosis of IBD; and second, to provide critical information for guiding the management of patients with known IBD.

Colonoscopy remains the method of choice to diagnose IBD, since the depiction of discrete morphologic signs, such as erythema, edema, granularity of the mucosa, small erosions, or scattered aphthoid ulcerations, can rarely be seen with conventional enteroclysis. They are also beyond the resolution of modern imaging techniques such as computed tomography (CT) or magnetic resonance imaging (MRI). Furthermore, ileo-colonoscopy allows biopsy specimens to be obtained for histologic investigation, underscoring its central role as the primary imaging modality in the diagnostic work-up of IBD.

Diagnosis

During the primary diagnostic step, patients with suspected IBD will be assigned to one of the two major chronic inflammatory diseases of the bowel: ulcerative colitis (UC) or Crohn's disease (CD). The key information required to optimize therapy for each disease is based on different factors, but localization, extent, and severity of bowel inflammation are crucial for both entities.

Until recently, this information was mainly obtained through barium studies and colonoscopy, which have been considered the gold standard in IBD imaging [1]. However, in CD, knowledge of the extraluminal manifestations of disease – including fistulae or abscesses – is pivotal for good patient management. Sepsis due to internal fistulae and abscesses was, in the 1970s, the most frequent cause of death related to CD [2]. Colonoscopy and enteroclysis provide little or no information on this extraluminal dimension.

Dramatic improvements in cross-sectional imaging (helical CT, MRI, and ultrasound) have led to a paradigm shift in the follow-up of patients with CD. Colonoscopy, small-bowel follow-through, enteroclysis, and barium enemas have been replaced by transabdominal bowel sonography (TABS), helical-CT enteroclysis (HCTE), and MR enteroclysis (MRE), all of which refine the standards of intestinal imaging in CD. These methods do not detect the morphologic signs of IBD as seen by colonoscopy, but display various degrees of bowel-wall thickening, contrast enhancement, and the extraluminal dimension of CD. This chapter highlights these imaging methods, specifically with regard to the management of CD, and discusses recent techniques and future trends.

Ultrasound

Over the past 2 decades, ultrasound has been recognized and evaluated as an emerging imaging modality to identify bowel-wall thickening in IBD [3]. During the late 1980s and early 1990s, the interest and skill in this novel, noninvasive imaging method grew [4].

TABS was tested for its accuracy in establishing the primary diagnosis, differentiating between the different forms of IBD, and evaluating the activity and extent of disease [5–7]. Technological improvements finally provided higher spatial and temporal resolution, allowing the discrimination of different bowel loops and bowel-wall layers. TABS is an inexpensive and radiation-free method that does not need bowel preparation; moreover, patients are allowed to have a small meal before TABS in order to provide some luminal distension. TABS not only identifies bowel-wall thickening of diseased loops, but also gives valid information on the presence of complications such as fistulae, abscesses, and strictures [8]. The real-time mode enables investigation of bowel motion, peristalsis, and the various degrees of obstruction. The procedure is pain free, noninvasive, and well tolerated by patients.

The downside of TABS is significant interobserver variation and lack of standardized image documentation. In addition, some parts of the abdomen are not easily visualized, such as ileal or distal colonic segments within the lower pelvis. Visibility in obese patients is limited in general.

The clinical impact of TABS

Bowel-wall thickening is the key sonographic feature in IBD. Normal bowel-wall segments measure between 1 mm and 2 mm, and inflammation results in thickening of intestinal segments. On cross-section, the inflamed bowel wall is recognized as a so-called "target sign lesion" (see **Figure 1**), in which various mucosal layers can be discriminated. The thicker the bowel wall, the narrower the bowel lumen. Therefore, bowel-wall thickening relates to the degree of bowel obstruction, and TABS is an excellent method for detecting strictures [9].

Although bowel-wall thickening does not correlate with clinical or biochemical markers of disease activity [10], the degree of bowel-wall thickening is thought to relate to the accumulation of chronic inflammatory changes. Different patterns of wall stratification do not appear to be related to clinical activity [11].

Power Doppler ultrasound technology and/or the use of intravenous ultrasound contrast media allow quantification of the vascular dimension of bowel-wall thickening [12,13]. Again, no

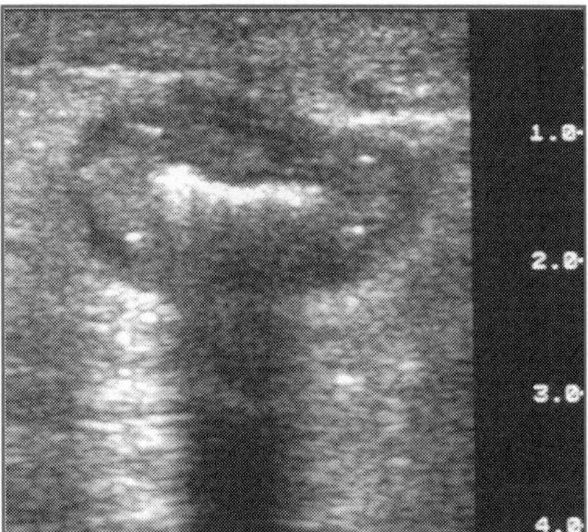

Figure 1. Transabdominal bowel sonography (TABS) of a definite Crohn's lesion with typical bowel-wall thickening (5–6 mm). Note the loss of strata between the mucosal and muscular layers. The bowel lumen is collapsed and shows hyperechoic content (most likely to be air).

relationship to clinical disease activity has been shown in CD. Interestingly, in UC, the degree of vascularization is higher in active disease [13]. The same technology has also been used to measure blood flow in close proximity to fistulae [14]. Whether vascularization of internal fistulae is a primary (fistula formation following tracks of pre-existing vessels) or secondary effect (fistulae induce neovascularization) has not been clarified [14,15].

For the gastroenterologist who sees IBD patients, TABS should be considered as important as echocardiography is for the cardiologist. The beauty of TABS lies in a combination of factors: it is readily available, with no need for bowel preparation, and is radiation-free, noninvasive, and very helpful for clinical decision-making, specifically in acutely ill patients. The dynamic nature of TABS enables the evaluation of bowel motility. The anatomic location of a partial or complete obstruction can be identified, and, in minor cases of obstruction, the functional degree of obstruction can be evaluated after a test meal.

Although 90% of TABS is performed in patients with CD, this technique can also give important information for the management of patients with UC. In those with active colitis, drug therapy depends on the extent of colonic disease involvement (left-sided colitis versus extended or pancolitis). Because the extent of colonic inflammation may vary between different flares, this information is relevant to patient management, and can be easily obtained through TABS.

Cross-sectional imaging

HCTE and MRE have emerged as the most important imaging techniques for evaluating the small intestine in CD for the following reasons: they are noninvasive, fast, well tolerated, widely accepted, and their accuracy in detecting the intramural and intraperitoneal extent of disease is excellent [16–19].

Helical-CT enteroclysis

HCTE is a relatively new imaging modality, which combines the advantages of conventional small-bowel enteroclysis (distension of the small bowel) with those of helical-CT (speed, resolution, volumetric data set, optimal utilization of the contrast media bolus) [19]. HCTE permits excellent morphologic evaluation of inflamed bowel walls, and has the potential to provide important additional information about any possible extraintestinal or extraperitoneal extension of the disease. In particular, the extent of inflammatory bowel-wall thickening, the presence or absence of a prestenotic dilatation, and extraintestinal manifestation provide important information (see **Figure 2**). Thus, a wide spectrum of abnormalities is seen with HCTE.

Small-bowel abnormalities and complications in CD (eg, fistulae or abscesses), which have a strong impact on clinical management, can be detected particularly well. Additional HCTE findings in IBD, such as fibrofatty proliferation or enlarged lymph nodes (mesenteric lymphadenitis), may add information to a patient's evaluation, but rarely change the clinical management.

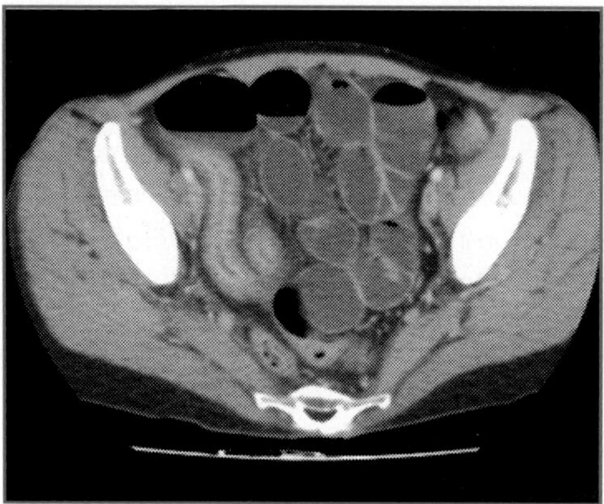

Figure 2. Helical-computed tomography enteroclysis (HCTE) image of ileitis in Crohn's disease showing a marked thickening of the bowel wall and increased enhancement after intravenous contrast media injection. The lumen is narrowed, but no prestenotic dilatation is found in this patient.

These features may indicate acute exacerbation of the inflammatory disease, but this is speculative and requires evaluation in future studies.

The influence of CT on the management of patients with IBD has been reported by Fishman et al [17]. They showed that clinical decisions were changed in 28% of patients who underwent conventional CT. HCTE expands the utility of CT in the management of patients with IBD, because the helical-CT mode provides improved image resolution along the z-axis, and offers excellent soft-tissue discrimination due to timely utilization of the injected contrast media.

Helical-CT provides volumetric data acquisition within a single breath-hold, thereby setting new standards in the depiction of sinus tracks, small fistulae, or peri-intestinal abscesses, and in the delineation of extraluminal involvement. The improved quality of 2D and 3D reconstructions may contribute to a better understanding of complex anatomical relationships, such as entero-enteral fistulae. An additional boost in resolution and sensitivity is expected with the widespread introduction of the new generation of CT scanners (multidetector row scanners).

Disadvantages of HCTE

The disadvantages of HCTE are the use of ionizing radiation and – compared with conventional double-contrast examinations – the lack of any dynamic information. Thus, differentiation between peristalsis and skip lesions may be difficult, and requires some experience.

Magnetic resonance enteroclysis

Due to its high inherent soft-tissue contrast, multiplanar capabilities, and use of nonionizing radiation, MRE is having an increasing impact on the diagnostic evaluation of IBD patients [21,22]. Technical improvements in hardware (phased-array coils, gradients) and software (better fat suppression, faster sequences, respiratory triggering) have helped to overcome "MRI-specific" limitations for imaging the gastrointestinal tract, such as low signal to noise ratio, and excessive motion artifacts resulting from peristalsis and respiration [23]. Indeed, MRE has become the most promising imaging modality in evaluating gastrointestinal diseases [24].

Like HCTE, MRE depicts thickened bowel loops, and illustrates both intestinal and extraintestinal abnormalities in CD (see **Figure 3**). The coronal plane provides a quick and reliable overview of the extent of disease; in particular, skip lesions are easily depicted. In addition, multiple imaging planes afford an improved depiction of the relationship between fistulae and adjacent organs.

Although MR machines are widely available, MRE is currently only performed in specialized centers. This is probably due to a general lack of experience in gastrointestinal MRI, and the fact that MRE is more time consuming (due to patient preparation and the number of sequences required) than a standard MR examination (eg, head, spine, or knee).

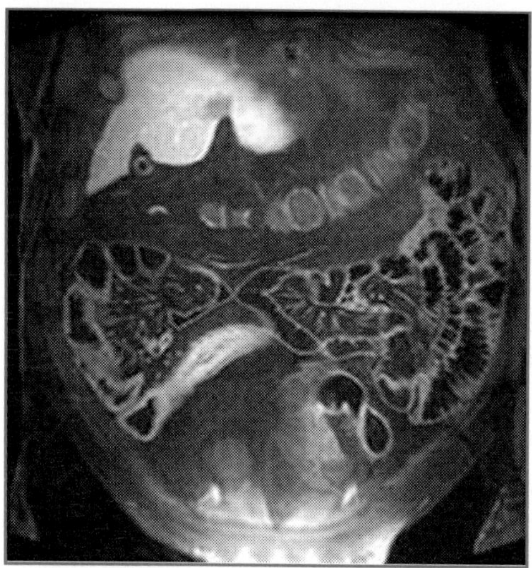

Figure 3. Coronal T1-weighted magnetic resonance enteroclysis image after intravenous contrast administration and fat suppression technique showing the extent of the diseased and thickened small bowel in a Crohn's disease patient. (Courtesy of Th. Lauenstein, University of Essen, Germany.)

At this point, HCTE is the imaging method of choice in patients with complicated CD, because the spatial resolution is higher with CT than with MR (ie, fistulae and sinus tracts are easier to depict). The bigger field of view used in MRE decreases the voxel size, and therefore the spatial resolution. However, the lack of ionizing radiation in MRE is particularly important, given that many patients with IBD are young. Comparative studies of MRE and HCTE are in progress.

Critical requirements for HCTE and MRE

The quality and accuracy of HCTE and MRE examinations are highly dependent on the distension of the bowel loops. Adequately distended bowel loops are crucial to enable depiction of stenotic segments, and to allow an accurate assessment of either segmental or diffuse circumferential inflammatory bowel-wall thickening [4]. In principle, a satisfying distension of the bowel loops can be achieved in two ways:

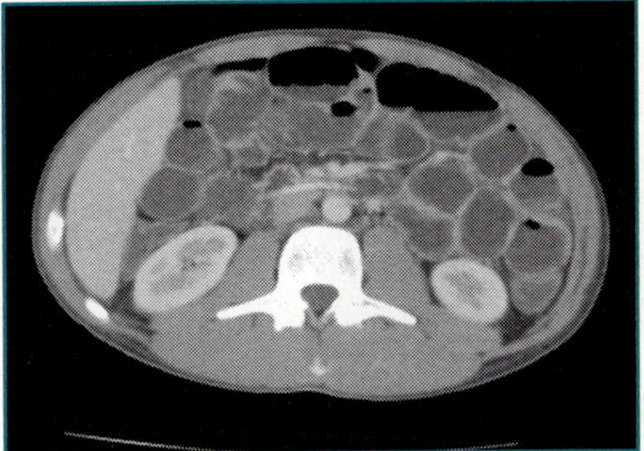

Figure 4. Helical-computed tomography enteroclysis (HCTE) image demonstrating the excellent distension of a normal small bowel after administration of methylcellulose via a nasoenteric tube.

- administration of fluid (eg, methylcellulose, dilute barium solution) via a nasoenteric tube, which usually provides adequate filling of the small intestine (see **Figure 4**)

- drinking of large amounts of fluid over a period of about 4 hours (eg, diluted gadolinium, iron-based suspensions, mannitol)

Recent reports stress the comfort and higher acceptance by patients of the second option [20]. Disadvantages of this method include possibly inadequate filling of the bowel loops, that it is more time consuming, and that vomiting may occur during the procedure because of the extensive filling of the stomach.

Pneumocolon-CT and CT/MR colonography

Filling and distension of the large bowel can be inadequate with both HCTE and MRE. Alternative imaging methods to evaluate the large bowel wall have been developed using helical-CT after distension of the large bowel with air or carbon dioxide via a rectal tube: this is known as "pneumocolon-CT". Patients prefer carbon dioxide as a distension medium, because it causes less pain than room air. Gas filling affords high quality views of the distended colon wall (see **Figure 5**).

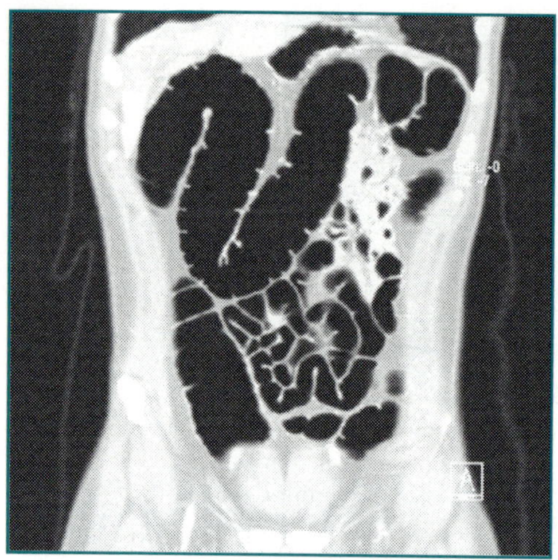

Figure 5. Coronal multislice-computed tomography (CT) image after perianal application of carbon dioxide (pneumocolon-CT). Images are usually evaluated in a "lung" window to enable better delineation of the inner contour of the large-bowel wall.

Pneumocolon-CT is as good as HCTE for imaging extracolonic complications. However, the small-bowel loops are usually collapsed and hence difficult to discriminate with pneumocolon-CT. Using 3D software, fly-through images can be generated (CT/MR colonography); but, the prolonged postprocessing time and need for high-end workstations limit applications of these methods to academic or specialized institutions.

Wireless capsule endoscopy

Discrete mucosal pathologies of the small intestine are notoriously difficult to diagnose. The resolution of both conventional barium studies and cross-sectional imaging methods is inadequate for detecting erythema, edema, or single aphthous lesions in the small bowel. Wireless capsule endoscopy, which was originally developed for small-bowel investigations in patients with obscure intestinal bleeding [25,26], is a new method for imaging patients with IBD.

This novel technology allows a pain- and radiation-free investigation of the small bowel, with excellent image quality. A single-use, wireless capsule holding a small videochip, transmitter, and battery is swallowed by the patient. The video images are taken continuously and data are sent to a small portable device and recorded. After the investigation, the data are transferred to a computer system, and the images are analyzed on a monitor by a physician. The average small-bowel transit time of the capsule is 3.5–4 hours. In healthy individuals, the capsule is finally passed with the stool within 24–48 hours.

Advantages

High patient tolerability adds to the excellent image quality and sensitivity of this new method. The video capsule endoscope has been shown to be superior to small-bowel radiography in the evaluation of various small-bowel diseases, including suspected CD [27]. Recently, data have been collected from patients with suspected small-bowel CD, and wireless capsule endoscopy was shown to be a superior diagnostic tool to barium follow-through or CT scans [28,29]. However, limitations, such as difficulties in interpreting potentially nonspecific findings, mean that this system requires further assessment. Furthermore, this method can only be used in patients without intestinal strictures.

Imaging of the pelvic floor

A total of 10%–30% of CD patients suffer from perianal disease [30]. Clinical management relies on knowledge of the morphology and anatomic location of fistulous tracts, and on information about perineal abscesses. Awareness of the exact topographic relationship between fistulae or abscesses and the pelvic floor is mandatory before surgery. Thus, highly accurate diagnostic imaging is desirable to obtain a detailed delineation of the lesions.

MRI

MRI has become the method of choice to illustrate the pelvic floor in IBD [31,32]. Most other imaging modalities (CT in particular)

	Primary diagnosis	Follow-up	
		Crohn's disease	Ulcerative colitis
Ileocolonoscopy with biopsy	+++	+	+++
Small-bowel enteroclysis	+	+	–
Transabdominal ultrasound	+	+++	++
HCT enteroclysis	+	+++	–
MR enteroclysis	+	+++	–
Pneumocolon CT	+	+++	+
Wireless capsule endoscopy	++	+	–
MRI of pelvic floor (EUS)	–	++	–

Table 1. Imaging in IBD. CT: computerized tomography; EUS: endoscopic ultrasound; HCT: helical computerized tomography; MR: magnetic resonance; MRI: magnetic resonance imaging. +: reasonable to use; –: not recommended.

cannot compete with MRI, and therefore should only be used in special cases (eg, where MRI is contraindicated). Fistulography should no longer be used.

Transanal endoscopic ultrasound

Transanal endoscopic ultrasound (EUS) is an inexpensive alternative to MRI [33]. EUS provides visualization of the anal canal and sphincter muscles. However, this method lacks depth penetration, and is therefore less suitable for extensive, deep fistulous tracts or abscesses.

As with TABS, EUS depends on the skill of the operator. The technical success rate of EUS is also limited by strictures of the anal canal. Moreover, in the event of local inflammatory changes, the examination may be very painful. In any case where surgery is considered, MRI is the method of choice.

Table 1 summarizes the available imaging techniques and their recommendations for use.

Functional imaging of IBD

Positron emission tomography (PET) with fluorine 18-labeled fluoro-2-deoxy-D-glucose (FDG) is a functional imaging method used to detect abnormalities in glucose metabolism in a variety of disorders, ranging from neurologic diseases to oncology. Several studies have indicated a role for PET in detecting areas of chronic inflammation [34–37].

FDG uptake increases in cells with high glycolytic rates, such as inflamed tissue, leading to accumulation of FDG-6-phospate. This increased glucose consumption allows visualization of inflammatory foci. Three reports have indicated a potential use for this procedure in localizing inflamed bowel segments in patients with CD [38–40]. PET imaging has proven superior to immunoscintigraphy [40]. Even more interestingly, PET identifies hot spots in areas that appear macroscopically normal during colonoscopy – possibly indicating that histologic inflammation can occur independent of ulceration. PET may also help to determine inflammatory activity within strictures, though more data are needed.

Future trends

TABS is the primary imaging modality in the follow-up of patients with CD, and, in institutions where ultrasound is performed by gastroenterologists, TABS is best performed by the gastroenterologist who is in charge of IBD patients. MRE and HCTE represent complementary imaging methods that are mainly used when IBD-associated complications are suspected or TABS is not available.

Improvements in cross-sectional imaging

Availability of the new generation of multidetector CTs is increasing. An additional boost in resolution, coupled with imaging in axial and coronal planes with the same voxel size (thus enabling reconstruction of the original acquired data set in any

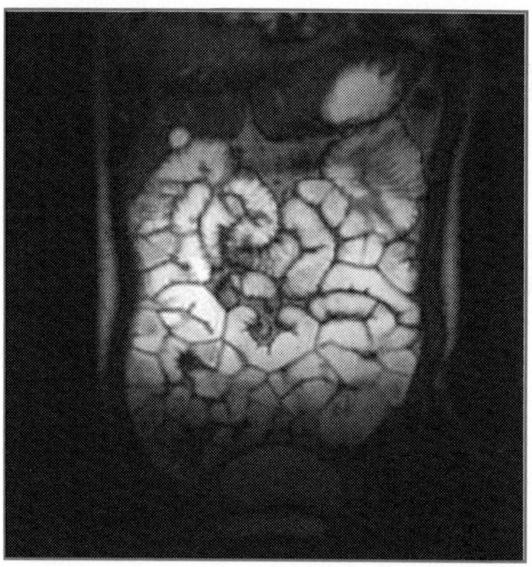

Figure 6. Coronal T2-weighted magnetic resonance enteroclysis image after oral administration of a distension medium. Excellent image quality and distension permit an improved evaluation of the intestine. (Courtesy of Th. Lauenstein, University of Essen, Germany.)

other plane – ie, sagittal, coronal, oblique, etc – with the same resolution), will expand the role of HCTE in the near future. MRE will prosper from continued improvements in coil and sequence design, and its resolution should increase to become comparable with HCTE. Furthermore, techniques for oral administration of distension media will begin to replace the use of nasoenteric tubes in routine examinations (see **Figure 6**).

Barium studies will undergo the same scrutiny as many other conventional x-ray methods, and will sometimes be completely replaced by cross-sectional imaging. HCTE and MRE have become the gold standard for small-bowel imaging (see **Figure 7**). It is conceivable that wireless capsule endoscopy will be implemented in the diagnostic evaluation of patients with suspected small-bowel disease and negative HCTE or MRE studies.

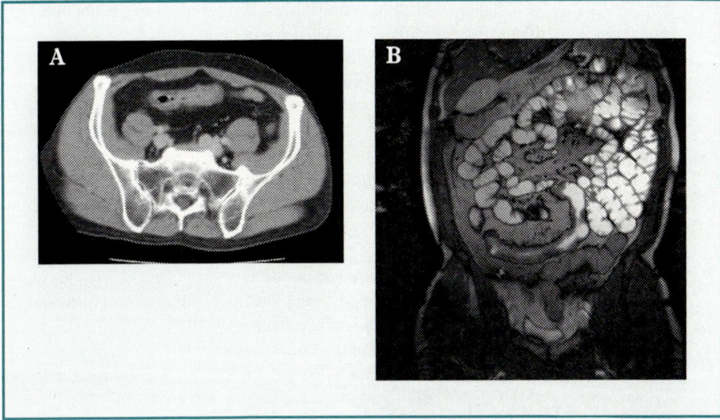

Figure 7. (**A**) Axial helical-computed tomography enteroclysis (HCTE) image showing marked thickening of the contrast-enhanced small-bowel wall in the terminal ileum. Note the prominent fatty tissue surrounding the inflamed bowel wall (fibrofatty proliferation) with displacement of the adjacent bowel loops. (**B**) Corresponding T2-weighted magnetic resonance enteroclysis (MRE) image in a coronal plane demonstrating thickening of the small-bowel wall. The coronal MR image gives an excellent overview of the entire bowel.

References

1. Herlinger HA. Modified technique for the double-contrast small bowel enema. *Gastrointest Radiol* 1978;2:201–7.
2. Farmer RG, Whelan G, Fazio VW. Long-term follow-up of patients with Crohn's disease. Relationship between the clinical pattern and prognosis. *Gastroenterology* 1985;88:1818–25.
3. Sonnenberg A, Erckenbrecht J, Peter P et al. Detection of Crohn's disease by ultrasound. *Gastroenterology* 1982;83:430–4.
4. Pedersen BH, Gronvall S, Dorph S et al. The value of dynamic ultrasound scanning in Crohn's disease. *Scand J Gastroenterol* 1986;21:969–72.
5. Meckler U, Caspary WF, Clement T et al. Sonography in Crohn disease – the conclusions of an experts' group. *Z Gastroenterol* 1991;29:355–9.
6. Worlicek H, Lutz H, Heyder N et al. Ultrasound findings in Crohn's disease and ulcerative colitis: a prospective study. *J Clin Ultrasound* 1987;15:153–63.
7. Maconi G, Imbesi V, Bianchi Porro G. Doppler ultrasound measurement of intestinal blood flow in inflammatory bowel disease. *Scand J Gastroenterol* 1996;31:590–3.
8. Gasche C, Moser G, Turetschek K et al. Transabdominal bowel sonography for the detection of intestinal complications in Crohn's disease. *Gut* 1999;44:112–7.
9. Parente F, Maconi G, Bollani S et al. Bowel ultrasound in assessment of Crohn's disease and detection of related small bowel strictures: a prospective comparative study versus x ray and intraoperative findings. *Gut* 2002;50:490–5.

10.   Maconi G, Parente F, Bollani S et al. Abdominal ultrasound in the assessment of extent and activity of Crohn's disease: clinical significance and implication of bowel wall thickening. *Am J Gastroenterol* 1996;91:1604–9.

11.   Futagami Y, Haruma K, Hata J et al. Development and validation of an ultrasonographic activity index of Crohn's disease. *Eur J Gastroenterol Hepatol* 1999; 11:1007–12.

12.   Di Sabatino A, Fulle I, Ciccocioppo R et al. Doppler enhancement after intravenous levovist injection in Crohn's disease. *Inflamm Bowel Dis* 2002;8:251–7.

13.   Heyne R, Rickes S, Bock P et al. Non-invasive evaluation of activity in inflammatory bowel disease by power Doppler sonography. *Z Gastroenterol* 2002;40:171–5.

14.   Maconi G, Sampietro GM, Russo A et al. The vascularity of internal fistulae in Crohn's disease: an in vivo power Doppler ultrasonography assessment. *Gut* 2002;50:496–500.

15.   Oberhuber G, Stangl PC, Vogelsang H et al. Significant association of strictures and internal fistula formation in Crohn's disease. *Virchows Arch* 2000;437:293–7.

16.   Orel SG, Rubesin SE, Jones B et al. Computed tomography vs barium studies in the acutely symptomatic patient with Crohn disease. *J Comput Assist Tomogr* 1987; 11:1009–16.

17.   Fishman EK, Wolf EJ, Jones B et al. CT evaluation of Crohn's disease: effect on patient management. *Am J Roentgenol* 1987;148:537–40.

18.   Gore RM. Cross-sectional imaging of inflammatory bowel disease. *Radiol Clin North Am* 1987;25:115–31.

19.   Bender GN, Maglinte D, Kloppel VR et al. CT enteroclysis: a superfluous diagnostic procedure or valuable when investigating small-bowel disease? *Am J Roentgenol* 1999;172:373–8.

20.   Papanikolaou N, Prassopoulos P, Grammatikakis J et al. Optimization of a contrast medium suitable for conventional enteroclysis, MR enteroclysis, and virtual MR enteroscopy. *Abdom Imaging* 2002;27:517–22.

21.   Gourtsoyiannis N, Papanikolaou N, Grammatikakis J et al. MR enteroclysis: technical considerations and clinical applications. *Eur Radiol* 2002;12:2651–8.

22.   Umschaden HW, Szolar D, Gasser J et al. Small-bowel disease: comparison of MR enteroclysis images with conventional enteroclysis and surgical findings. *Radiology* 2000;215:717–25.

23.   Paley MR, Ros PR. MRI of the gastrointestinal tract. *Eur Radiol* 1997;7:1387–97.

24.   Gourtsoyiannis N, Papanikolaou N, Grammatikakis J et al. MR imaging of the small bowel with a true-FISP sequence after enteroclysis with water solution. *Invest Radiol* 2000;35:707–11.

25.   Ell C, Remke S, May A et al. The first prospective controlled trial comparing wireless capsule endoscopy with push enteroscopy in chronic gastrointestinal bleeding. *Endoscopy* 2002;34:685–9.

26.   Lewis BS, Swain P. Capsule endoscopy in the evaluation of patients with suspected small intestinal bleeding: results of a pilot study. *Gastrointest Endosc* 2002;56:349–53.

27.   Costamagna G, Shah SK, Riccioni ME et al. A prospective trial comparing small bowel radiographs and video capsule endoscopy for suspected small bowel disease. *Gastroenterology* 2002;123:999–1005.

28.   Eliakim R, Fischer D, Suissa A et al. Wireless capsule video endoscopy is a superior diagnostic tool in comparison to barium follow through and computerised tomography in patients with suspected Crohn's disease. *Eur J Gastroenterol Hepatol* 2003 (in press).

29.   Fireman Z, Mahajna E, Broide E et al. Diagnosing small bowel Crohn's disease with wireless capsule endoscopy. *Gut* 2003;52:390–2.

30.   Rankin GB, Watts HD, Melnyk CS et al. National Cooperative Crohn's Disease Study: extraintestinal manifestations and perianal complications. *Gastroenterology* 1979; 77:914–20.

31. Hussain SM, Stoker J, Schouten WR et al. Fistula in ano:endoanal sonography versus endoanal MR imaging in classification. *Radiology* 1996;200:475–81.

32. Jenss H, Starlinger M, Skaleij M. Magnetic resonance imaging in perianal Crohn's disease. *Lancet* 1992;340:1286.

33. Schratter-Sehn AU, Lochs H, Vogelsang H et al. Endoscopic ultrasonography versus computed tomography in the differential diagnosis of perianorectal complications in Crohn's disease. *Endoscopy* 1993;25:582–6.

34. Goo JM, Im JG, Do KH et al. Pulmonary tuberculoma evaluated by means of FDG PET: findings in 10 cases. *Radiology* 2000;216:117–21.

35. Ichiya Y, Kuwabara Y, Sasaki M et al. FDG-PET in infectious lesions: the detection and assessment of lesion activity. *Ann Nucl Med* 1996;10:185–91.

36. Zhuang H, Pourdehnad M, Lambright ES et al. Dual time point 18F-FDG PET imaging for differentiating malignant from inflammatory processes. *J Nucl Med* 2001;42:1412–7.

37. Zhuang H, Alavi A. 18-fluorodeoxyglucose positron emission tomographic imaging in the detection and monitoring of infection and inflammation. *Semin Nucl Med* 2002;32:47–59.

38. Bicik I, Bauerfeind P, Breitbach T et al. Inflammatory bowel disease activity measured by positron-emission tomography. *Lancet* 1997;350:262.

39. Skehan SJ, Issenman R, Mernagh J et al. 18F-fluorodeoxyglucose positron tomography in diagnosis of paediatric inflammatory bowel disease. *Lancet* 1999;354:836–7.

40. Neurath MF, Vehling D, Schunk K et al. Noninvasive assessment of Crohn's disease activity: a comparison of 18F-fluorodeoxyglucose positron emission tomography, hydromagnetic resonance imaging, and granulocyte scintigraphy with labeled antibodies. *Am J Gastroenterol* 2002;97:1978–85.

6

Probiotics: rationale, challenges, and scope

Fergus Shanahan

Introduction

The development of inflammatory bowel diseases (IBD) – Crohn's disease (CD) and ulcerative colitis (UC) – involves a convergence of three elements in the pathogenesis: genetic susceptibility, immune activation or dysregulation, and environmental trigger(s) [1,2]. Only one component of the pathogenesis – the host's immune response – is targeted by most current therapeutic strategies.

Despite remarkable advances, the efficacy of immunomodulatory agents is limited to a subset of patients, requires increased vigilance for toxicity, and is associated with considerable cost. Targeting the environmental contribution to IBD may enable a more comprehensive, and sustained, therapeutic response.

Gastroenterologists are fully aware of the importance of resident bacteria in human disease. For decades, the management of peptic ulcer disease consisted of modifying the host response by suppression or neutralization of gastric acid. When the contribution of *Helicobacter pylori* to the pathogenesis of peptic ulcer disease was discovered, lasting therapy was accomplished. In CD and UC, the relationship between the enteric flora and disease pathogenesis may be more complex and subtle.

Although a transmissible infectious agent might contribute to the pathogenesis and act as a cofactor in IBD, these diseases appear to reflect an abnormal immune response to normal flora, rather than a normal host response to abnormal flora [1–4]. Because the composition of the commensal flora varies in its proinflammatory capacity, modification of enteric bacterial populations has emerged as a potential therapeutic strategy in IBD.

While the use of antibiotics is an obvious approach to modifying the indigenous flora, it suffers from major disadvantages, such as lack of selection, risk of toxicity, and potential development of bacterial resistance; furthermore, antibiotics are not suitable for long-term use.

This chapter focuses on probiotic strategies. Probiotics are an attractive option because of their relative safety. However, optimal probiotic usage is limited by large gaps in our understanding of the normal flora, and by several potential clinical challenges and pitfalls.

Pathogenesis of IBD

Environmental triggers

An environmental contribution to the pathogenesis of IBD is highlighted by incomplete concordance rates for CD (<50%) and UC (<10%) in monozygotic twins [5]. Smoking is a confirmed risk factor, and appears to influence disease phenotype and severity in a subset of patients. However, the external and indigenous microbial environment is likely to exert the predominant influence on disease frequency.

Significant increases in the worldwide incidence and prevalence of IBD in recent decades cannot be accounted for on the basis of changes in population susceptibility genes over such a short period of time. A transmissible infectious agent, much like *H. pylori* in peptic disease, would be the simplest explanation for an environmental influence on the pathogenesis and changing epidemiology of IBD – but, while this hypothesis cannot be discounted, it is difficult to reconcile with certain clinical and epidemiologic observations.

Environmental conditions such as overcrowding, endemic parasitism, and poor sanitation, which should favor dispersal of a transmissible infectious agent, have the opposite effect in CD and exert an apparent protective influence [6,7]. In addition, there are no compelling data to indicate either horizontal or vertical transmission of CD or UC. In responsive patients, the therapeutic impact of long-term immune suppression is at variance with an infectious etiology. Although therapeutic antagonism of tumor necrosis factor (TNF)-α has been sufficient to pose a significant clinical risk of disseminated tuberculosis [8], it has not been linked with dissemination of *Mycobacterium paratuberculosis* or other pathogens claimed to be etiologic factors in IBD. While microbial DNA is detectable in the lesions of some patients with CD, it does not imply a cause-and-effect relationship, and may have a modifying influence on local cytokine profiles [9].

The environmental influence on the epidemiology and pathogenesis of IBD may relate to changes in immune perception of the microbial environment. Furthermore, genes that protect against infection in an unsanitary environment might, in effect, become susceptibility genes for IBD in developed countries [10]. For example, a survival advantage from genetically determined enhanced mucosal immunity to infection in developing countries might be a risk factor for immune-mediated disease when environmental and lifestyle conditions change.

As countries become more developed, the increasing prevalence of IBD has been paralleled by similar trends in other chronic inflammatory disorders, such as allergies, asthma, multiple sclerosis, and insulin-dependent diabetes mellitus [11]. It seems unlikely that environmental effects on the epidemiology of these conditions involve separate transmissible infections of multiple target end organs. A more plausible explanation may be that environmental factors act at the level of the immune system.

In common with other sensory systems, mucosal immune function requires appropriate input to promote learning, memory,

Factors that may influence mucosal immune education

- Improved sanitation and hygiene
- Life on concrete (reduced exposure to soil microbes in urban areas)
- Reduced consumption of fermented food products
- Increased consumption of semi-sterile food and beverages
- Decline in prevalence of *Helicobacter pylori*
- Decline in endemic parasitism
- Increased antibiotic usage
- Increased use of vaccinations
- Smaller family size
- Reduced or delayed exposure to mucosal infections

Table 1. Elements of modern lifestyle in developed societies that may influence mucosal immune education and represent a risk factor for inflammatory bowel diseases in genetically susceptible individuals.

and adaptation [12]. Mucosal immune development is incomplete at birth and continues to develop throughout childhood. Environmental contact with the intestinal commensal flora and with childhood infections determines the fine-tuning of T-cell repertoires and cytokine balance [13].

As countries develop and become industrialized, changes in lifestyle and environmental conditions may collectively represent a risk factor for IBD in genetically susceptible individuals (see **Table 1**). In this respect, the distinction between a commensal and a pathogen may be moot, depending on an individual's genetic constitution, and external and internal environmental exposure. Optimal mucosal immune function requires discriminatory accuracy and precise regulation to interpret the intestinal microbial environment. Generally, excessive immune reactivity against commensals is avoided, whilst the capacity for effective immune responses to episodic challenge with pathogens is retained. In contrast, anomalous interpretation or response to commensal and/or pathogenic bacterial signals from the lumen appears to be a fundamental risk factor for chronic IBD.

Health asset	Liability
• Mucosal defence – bacterial antagonism	• Conversion of some procarcinogens to carcinogens
• Production of nutrients, eg, short-chain fatty acids	• Induction of bacterial overgrowth syndromes
• Priming of mucosal immunity	• Opportunism and translocation
• Conversion of prodrugs to active metabolites, eg, sulfasalazine	• Essential ingredient for inflammatory bowel diseases
• Promotion of peristalsis	
• Synthesis of B and K vitamins	

Table 2. Enteric bacterial flora: health asset versus liability.

Modification of the intestinal flora

The indigenous enteric bacterial flora are critical for the normal development of the structure and function of the gut. Studies with germ-free animals, coupled with modern molecular techniques, show that the bacteria within the intestinal lumen exchange regulatory signals with the epithelium and subepithelial structures [14,15]. In most circumstances, the flora represents a health asset. However, in some instances, depending on genetic and other susceptibility factors, it represents a potential liability (see **Table 2**).

Strategies designed to promote the beneficial effects and offset any adverse influence of the flora in disease may open up new therapeutic opportunities. In IBD, several lines of observational and experimental evidence have implicated the flora as an essential ingredient in pathogenesis (see **Table 3**) [2,4].

Interestingly, the intestinal bacteria are not uniform in their capacity to drive the mucosal inflammatory response. Different bacterial species, particularly bacteroides and clostridial strains, have been specifically implicated in different animal models of IBD [4]. However, other commensals, such as *Lactobacillus* and *Bifidobacterium* species, have minimal proinflammatory capacity

Observational	Experimental
• Lesions in IBD tend to occur in areas of bowel with highest bacterial numbers	• Bacterial flora condition mucosal integrity and immune function
• Beneficial effect of diversion of fecal stream in CD; relapse is predictable with restoration of stream	• Reported efficacy of probiotics and antibiotics
• Development of pouchitis – in ulcerative colitis – after bacterial colonization of pouch	• Development of IBD, irrespective of the genetic defect, when murine models are colonized with commensals
• Immune reactivity to enteric bacteria is demonstrable in patients with IBD, and may reflect loss of tolerance to flora	• Induction of early lesions of CD by instillation of fecal material into excluded loops of bowel in susceptible subjects
• Patients with defective phagocytic microbicidal function, eg, glycogen storage disease type 1b, chronic granulomatous disease, and Hermansky–Pudlak syndrome, develop CD-like lesions that respond to antibiotics and treatment of the immune defect for bacterial products	• Identification of the *NOD2* (*CARD15*) susceptibility gene for CD. NOD2 proteins are intracytoplasmic receptors
• Abnormal host–flora interactions, possibly due to increased numbers of mucosal bacteria in CD	

Table 3. Evidence linking commensal flora with the pathogenesis of inflammatory bowel diseases (IBD). CD: Crohn's disease; NOD: nucleotide-binding oligomerization domain.

and are less likely to translocate from the lumen to the internal milieu [1,4]. For this reason, they are commonly selected as potential probiotics.

The virtual organ – human intestinal microflora

- Human intestinal flora comprises more bacteria than there are cells in the body
- Intestinal bacteria exceed the number of humans ever to have lived on the planet
- There are 1–2 kg of bacteria in the human gut
- Collective metabolic activity is tantamount to that of an organ the size of the liver
- The collective microbiome (multiple microbial genomes) is greater than the human genome

Table 4. The scale of the probiotic challenge.

Rationale for probiotic use

The previous section indicates that the rationale for therapeutic modification of the flora in IBD is derived primarily from the conditioning effects of the flora on mucosal integrity and immune function. From first principles, it may be argued that anything that can promote the microbial asset served by the normal flora, whilst offsetting any liabilities (see **Table 2**), has the potential to serve a health benefit. In addition, there is potential for probiotic strains to compete with or displace proinflammatory microbial stimuli or pathogenic organisms from the epithelial surface.

The probiotic challenge

When considering therapeutic modification of the gut flora, it is important to recognize that the bacteria occupying the length of the alimentary tract – from oral cavity to anus – represent an enormously complex ecosystem [3,17,18]. Some extraordinary statistics reveal the scale of the probiotic challenge, and why the intestinal microbiota can be likened to a virtual organ (see **Table 4**).

There are 400–500 bacterial species in the gut, at least half of which cannot be cultured at present, but are identifiable by molecular methods [19–21]. For this reason, comparatively little is known about the metabolic activity of intestinal bacteria. Molecular bacterial fingerprinting techniques suggest that the composition of the flora is generally stable – but individual – after weaning in infancy, although this appears to be subject to host genetic influences [21].

In contrast, environmental factors, such as sanitary or dietary variables, appear to exert their influence on the composition of the flora only at the early stages of gastrointestinal colonization, and are likely to determine the induction of bacterial enzymes and metabolic activity of the established flora [3,16,17]. The composition of the flora at the mucosal surface differs from that within the lumen and feces, with the ratio of anaerobes to aerobes being lower at mucosal surfaces.

In addition, the flora composition varies along the long axis of the bowel, with increasing complexity and variety from foregut to hindgut. The greatest gradient is found across the ileocecal valve, where there are approximately 1×10^8 bacteria/g of ileal content versus up to 1×10^{12} bacteria/g of colonic content [3,17]. It is evident that the selection of a given probiotic needs to take into consideration the viability and numbers of the probiotic strain, and their potential to occupy different microbial niches within the gut.

Selection criteria

Probiotics are biological control agents. A current operational definition encompasses "live micro-organisms which, when consumed in adequate amounts, confer a health benefit on the host" [22,23]. The emphasis here is on the live nature of the micro-organism. At present, there is no reliable *in vitro* predictor of *in vivo* efficacy of putative probiotics. The most commonly used probiotics are lactobacilli and bifidobacteria, though other bacteria, such as nonpathogenic *Escherichia coli*, and even nonbacterial organisms, such as *Saccharomyces boulardii*, have been used for probiotic effect.

In contrast, prebiotics are nondigestible food ingredients that beneficially affect the host by selectively stimulating the growth of bacterial species already established in the colon, and thus improve host health. These are usually of a polysaccharide or oligosaccharide nature.

The combination of probiotics and prebiotics is referred to as synbiotics. Each of these are also categorized as functional foods (foods or food components) that confer a beneficial effect beyond that of their nutritional content alone [24]. Some commentators have even declared that future consumer demand may require that all foods be functional.

The rapidly emerging field of functional foods, or nutraceuticals, is at the interface of the food and pharmaceutical industries. Understanding the molecular determinants and mechanisms of probiotic action will facilitate the development of novel therapies and may make it possible to shift from "bugs to drugs".

The Joint Food and Agricultural Organization of the United Nations and the World Health Organization have generated guidelines for probiotic strain identification and functional characterization [22,23]. These include properties such as acid and bile resistance, suitability for oral consumption, and survival during gastrointestinal transit. However, an ideal probiotic strain has not yet been identified for any indication.

There is a growing, but poorly regulated, commercial market in the area of functional foods and probiotics, which is often linked with tenuous or exaggerated claims made for their effectiveness in the lay press. Comprehensive comparisons of probiotic performance using different strains need to be completed in specific disease states. In addition, the impact of individual variations in the composition of host flora and the influence of indigenous bacterial metabolism on probiotic efficacy have yet to be determined.

Probiotics have been proposed for use in allergic, inflammatory, neoplastic, and infectious disorders. It seems unlikely that any single microbial agent would be equally suited to each of these diverse conditions.

Dosimetry

The dose range, frequency of administration, and optimal vehicle of delivery for different probiotics have not been settled conclusively. Probiotic product stability and its verification and regulation have not been standardized internationally. Furthermore, the effective dose of probiotics is likely to be influenced by survival during gastric transit, and possibly by the potential for colonization and multiplication within the colon.

Monitoring

In the absence of definitive data, current trials of probiotic maintenance therapy that are underway in Europe have incorporated a mechanism by which ingested probiotic organisms can be identified and quantified in excreted stools. This involves both conventional culture-dependent methods and molecular probes. In the case of *Lactobacillus salivarius* UCC118, a consistent profile of fecal levels of the probiotic after a 3-week feeding period has been demonstrated [25]. In addition, the kinetics of the probiotic's arrival at the terminal ileum – and, therefore, the ability of the organism to survive gastric acid, bile, and small-bowel transit – has been demonstrated [25]. While fecal analysis is a convenient method for confirming compliance during a therapeutic trial, and for demonstrating gastrointestinal survival and transit, the fecal flora may not be a true reflection of probiotic numbers in different microbial niches. This variability in microbial composition at different sites may also mean that a single probiotic will not be suited to different patients with CD, depending on the topographic distribution of the lesions.

Single strains or combinations

Until the mechanism of action of probiotics in different situations is clarified, the optimal therapeutic use of one or more strains cannot be conclusively determined. Combinations of strains might be a pragmatic strategy to encompass a range of indications and individual variations, but this assumes that the probiotic constituents of any combination are not mutually antagonistic. There is some experimental evidence to indicate that this may not be a valid assumption in the case of lactobacilli and bifidobacteria mixtures [26, O'Mahony et al., unpublished data].

Furthermore, as with all combinations of therapies, the activities of the individual components require definition of optimal usage before the combination can be routinely recommended. Probiotic research is still in its infancy, and there is much work to be done before it can be considered well established in modern evidence-based medicine.

Probiotics in practice

The role for probiotic strategies in IBD and non-IBD conditions such as atopy, infection, and cancer have been reviewed elsewhere [1,22,27]. Several investigators have confirmed the efficacy of probiotic feeding in animal models of IBD [28, 29]. The induction of remission in a patient with UC after implantation of exogenous normal flora using large volume retention enemas was described over a decade ago [30]. Despite this provocative report, microbial therapy in general – and probiotics in particular – have only recently attracted the attention of clinicians in the context of human IBD.

Trials in CD have deployed *Lactobacillus GG* [31], *S. boulardii* [32], and *E. coli* strain Nissle [33]. Results have been conflicting and confounded by the small size of the patient populations and differences in disease activity and distribution [34]. In UC, the nonpathogenic strain of *E. coli* Nissle appears to have efficacy equivalent to that of mesalazine [35,36].

However, the most compelling evidence for probiotics in IBD therapy reported a probiotic cocktail of eight bacterial strains in maintenance of remission of pouchitis [37]. It is clear that the promise of probiotics in IBD greatly exceeds the evidence for efficacy at present; more controlled trials are needed with strain–strain comparisons.

Mechanisms of action

It seems unlikely that a single mechanism of action is operative in the diversity of infectious, inflammatory, and atopic clinical conditions where probiotics have been reported to have clinical efficacy. In relation to host defense, probiotic activity may reflect competitive metabolic interactions, production of antimicrobials, and inhibition of adherence or translocation of pathogens. There is experimental evidence for each of these protective functions *in vitro* [4].

Indeed, novel antimicrobial bacteriocins have been identified by exploration of probiotic organisms [38], but the degree to which *in vitro* data can be extrapolated to *in vivo* settings is unclear. Other properties, such as an influence on mucosal barrier function, may underpin the beneficial effects reported for probiotics in atopy [39], and multiple mechanisms have been proposed to account for an anticancer effect [40].

In the context of IBD, anti-inflammatory probiotic effects may involve signaling with the epithelium and mucosal immune system. Since the indigenous commensal flora exert a regulatory influence on epithelial and subepithelial structures within the gut [15,16], it seems likely that probiotics have similar effects. Indeed, the molecular basis by which some nonpathogenic intestinal organisms counterbalance the epithelial responses to invasive bacteria has been explored at the level of cytokine transcription factors [41]. Transduction of bacterial signals into host immune responses is poorly understood, but nuclear factor (NF)-κB has emerged as a central regulator of epithelial responses to pathogens, such as invasive Salmonella [42,43]. In contrast, the inhibitory counter-regulatory factor to NF-κB (I-κB) seems to be exploited by some nonpathogenic components of the flora, which may attenuate proinflammatory responses by delaying the degradation of I-κB [41].

It is unlikely that probiotic bifidobacteria and lactobacilli use the same mechanism, and other signal transduction pathways are likely to emerge to account for their anti-inflammatory effects. In addition to epithelial and cytokine responses, a probiotic impact on mucosal regulatory T cells is currently under scrutiny (Shanahan et al., unpublished data).

Probiotics or other food-grade organisms can be modified or engineered to exhibit specific functional activity, such as the delivery of anti-inflammatory cytokines or other biologically active molecules to the gut. This has already been accomplished with *Lactococcus lactis* engineered to secrete interleukin (IL)-10, where the local production of IL-10 within the gut was found to be as efficacious as corticosteroid therapy in two animal models of IBD [44].

The potential applications of this strategy are intriguing, though public health and other safety concerns need to be resolved before it can be applied to humans [45].

Future directions

Probiotics hold great promise for IBD therapy, but this field of research is still developmental. Analyses of the potential role of probiotics in modern medicine have ranged from dubious [46], to reserved [47,48], to enthusiastic [49]. Several gaps in our knowledge and potential pitfalls persist [50]. These can only be resolved with better characterization of individual strains, clarification of mechanisms of action in different settings, and carefully controlled clinical trials.

Probiotic performance should be defined in terms of the health benefit that is required, eg, anti-inflammatory, anti-infective, or both. Furthermore, in complex disorders such as IBD, there may be subset-specific indications requiring strain-specific prescriptions. Problems with probiotic usage have already been alluded to, and particular issues that need to be addressed are listed in **Table 5**.

Challenges and confounding variables with probiotic strategies

- Lack of fidelity of *in vitro* assays to predict *in vivo* probiotic performance
- Optimal strain selection criteria not defined according to disease indications
- Optimal dose and delivery vehicle not confirmed
- Poor verification and regulation of probiotic product stability
- Lack of rigorous strain–strain comparisons of probiotic performance
- Individual probiotic strains may not be equally suited to each disease indication
- Different probiotics may be required for different microbial niches, with attendant implications for variations in disease distribution in Crohn's disease
- Some probiotic combinations may be antagonistic

Table 5. Challenges and confounding variables with probiotic strategies.

There is the difficult regulatory issue of whether probiotics should be treated as food supplements, drugs, or both. The appeal of probiotic therapy is their safety in comparison with drugs. However, the use of probiotics by healthy individuals and the therapeutic application of probiotics in high dosages to individuals with gastrointestinal disease are distinct issues that may require separate regulatory surveillance. Results of studies showing probiotic performance in any given clinical setting cannot be extrapolated to another disease indication, and will require separate assessment.

It is likely that the definition of probiotics will continue to evolve and will almost certainly embrace genetically modified organisms in the future. Once the molecular determinants of probiotic action are understood, it may be possible to shift from bugs to drugs. Indeed, the immunomodulatory properties of bacterial DNA have already shown therapeutic potential in the context of mucosal inflammation [51].

Acknowledgements

The author is supported in part by the Health Research Board of Ireland, the Higher Education Authority of Ireland, and the European Union (PROGID QLK-2000-00563). The author is affiliated with a multidepartmental university campus company (Alimentary Health Ltd, Ireland), which investigates host–flora interactions, and the therapeutic manipulation of these interactions in various human and animal disorders. The content of this chapter was neither influenced nor constrained by this fact.

References

1. Shanahan F. Inflammatory bowel disease: immunodiagnostics, immunotherapeutics, and ecotherapeutics. *Gastroenterology* 2001;120:622–35.
2. Shanahan F. Crohn's disease. *Lancet* 2002;359:62–9.
3. Bengmark S. Ecological control of the gastrointestinal tract. The role of probiotic flora. *Gut* 1998;42:2–7.
4. Shanahan F. Probiotics in inflammatory bowel disease: is there a scientific rationale? *Inflamm Bowel Dis* 2000;6:107–15.
5. Tysk C, Lindberg E, Jarnerot G et al. Ulcerative colitis and Crohn's disease in an unselected population of monozygotic and dizygotic twins. A study of heritability and the influence of smoking. *Gut* 1988;29:990–6.
6. Gent AE, Hellier MD, Grace RH et al. Inflammatory bowel disease and domestic hygiene in infancy. *Lancet* 1994;343:766–7.
7. Elliott DE, Urban JF Jr, Argo CK et al. Does the failure to acquire helminthic parasites predispose to Crohn's disease? *FASEB J* 2000;14:1848–55.
8. Keane J, Gershon S, Wise RP et al. Tuberculosis associated with infliximab, a tumor necrosis factor alpha-neutralising agent. *N Engl J Med* 2001;345:1098–104.
9. Ryan P, Bennett MW, Aarons S et al. PCR detection of Mycobacterium paratuberculosis in Crohn's disease granulomas isolated by laser capture microdissection. *Gut* 2002;51:665–70.
10. Taylor KD, Rotter JI, Yang H. Genetics of inflammatory bowel disease. In: Targan SR, Shanahan F, Karp LC, editors. *Inflammatory Bowel Disease: From Bench to Bedside*, 2nd Edition. Dordrecht: Kluwer Academic Publishers, 2003:21–65.
11. Bach JF. The effect of infections on susceptibility to autoimmune and allergic diseases. *N Engl J Med* 2002;347:911–20.
12. Shanahan F. Nutrient tasting and signaling mechanisms in the gut V. Mechanisms of immunologic sensation of intestinal contents. *Am J Physiol Gastrointest Liver Physiol* 2000;278:G191–6.
13. Rook GA, Stanford JL. Give us this day our daily germs. *Immunol Today* 1998;19:113–6.
14. Midtvedt T. Microbial functional activities. In: Hanson LA, Yolken RH, editors. *Probiotics, Other Nutritional Factors, and Intestinal Microflora* (Nestle Nutrition Workshop Series, v. 42). Lippincott Williams & Wilkins Publishers, 1999:79–96.

15. Gordon JI, Hooper LV, McNevin MS et al. Epithelial cell growth and differentiation. III. Promoting diversity in the intestine: conversations between the microflora, epithelium, and diffuse GALT. *Am J Physiol* 1997;273(3 Pt.1):G565–70.

16. Hooper LV, Gordon JI. Commensal host-bacterial relationships in the gut. *Science* 2001;292:1115–8.

17. Berg RD. The indigenous gastrointestinal microflora. *Trends Microbiol* 1996;4:430–5.

18. Bocci V. The neglected organ: bacterial flora has a crucial immunostimulatory role. *Perspect Biol Med* 1992;35:251–60.

19. Vaughan EE, Schut F, Heilig HG et al. A molecular view of the intestinal ecosystem. *Curr Issues Intest Microbiol* 2000;1:1–12.

20. Akkermans ADL, Zoetendal EG, Favier CF et al. Temperature and denaturing gradient gel electrophoresis analysis of 16S rRNA from human faecal samples. *Bioscience Microflora* 2000;19:93–8.

21. Van de Merwe JP, Stegeman JH, Hazenberg MP. The resident faecal flora is determined by genetic characteristics of the host. Implications for Crohn's disease? *Antonie Van Leeuwenhoek* 1983;49:119–24.

22. Report of a Joint FAO/WHO Expert Consultation. Health and nutritional properties of probiotics in food including powder milk and live lactic acid bacteria, Argentina, 2001. Available at: URL: http://www.who.int/fsf/Documents/Powder_milk_report.pdf

23. Guidelines for the evaluation of probiotics in food. Joint FAO/WHO Working Group Report on Drafting Guidelines for the Evaluation of Probiotics in Food, London Ontario, Canada, 2002. Available at: URL: http://www.agr.gc.ca/food/nff/pdfdocs/probiotics.pdf.

24. Shanahan F, McCarthy J. Functional foods and probiotics: time for gastroenterologists to embrace the concept. *Curr Gastroenterol Rep* 2000;2:345–6.

25. Collins JK, Murphy L, Morrissey D et al. A randomised controlled trial of a probiotic Lactobacillus strain in healthy adults: assessment of its delivery, transit, and influence on microbial flora and enteric immunity. *Microb Ecol Health Dis* 2002;14:81–9.

26. Murphy LM, Byrne FR, Collins JK et al. Evaluation and characterisation of probiotic therapy in the CD45RH (hi) transfer model of colitis. *Gastroenterology* 1999;116:780A (Abstr.)

27. Dunne C, Shanahan F. Role of probiotics in the treatment of intestinal infections and inflammation. *Curr Opin Gastroenterol* 2002;18:40–5.

28. Madsen KL, Doyle JS, Jewell LD et al. Lactobacillus species prevents colitis in interleukin 10 gene-deficient mice. *Gastroenterology* 1999;116:1107–14.

29. O'Mahony L, Feeney M, O'Halloran S et al. Probiotic impact on microbial flora, inflammation and tumor development in IL-10 knockout mice. *Aliment Pharmacol Ther* 2001;15:1219–25.

30. Bennet JD, Brinkman M. Treatment of ulcerative colitis by implantation of normal colonic flora. *Lancet* 1989;1:164.

31. Prantera C, Scribano ML, Falasco G et al. Ineffectiveness of probiotics in preventing recurrence after curative resection for Crohn's disease: a randomised controlled trial with Lactobacillus GG. *Gut* 2002;51:405–9.

32. Guslandi M, Mezzi G, Sorghi M et al. Sacharomyces boulardii in maintenance treatment of Crohn's disease. *Dig Dis Sci* 2000;45:1462–4.

33. Malchow HA. Crohn's disease and Escherichia coli. A new approach in therapy to maintain remission of colonic Crohn's disease? *J Clin Gastroenterol* 1997;25:653–8.

34. Hamilton-Miller JMT. A review of clinical trials of probiotics in the management of inflammatory bowel disease. *Infect Dis Rev* 2001;3:83-7.

35. Kruis W, Schütz E, Fric P et al. Double-blind comparison of an oral *Escherichia coli* preparation and mesalazine in maintaining remission of ulcerative colitis. *Aliment Pharmacol Ther* 1997;11:853–8.

36. Rembacken BJ, Snelling AM, Hawkey PM et al. Non-pathogenic *Escherichia coli* versus mesalazine for the treatment of ulcerative colitis: a randomised trial. *Lancet* 1999;354:635–9.

37. Gionchietti P, Rizzello F, Venturi A et al. Oral bacteriotherapy as maintenance treatment in patients with chronic pouchitis: a double-blind, placebo-controlled trial. *Gastroenterology* 2000;119:305–9.

38. Flynn S, van Sinderen D, Thornton GM et al. Characterization of the genetic locus responsible for the production of ABP-118, a novel bacteriocin produced by the probiotic bacterium *Lactobacillus salivarius* subsp. salivarius UCC118. *Microbiology* 2002;148:973–84.

39. Isolauri E, Majamaa H, Arvola T et al. *Lactobacillus casei* strain GG reverses increased intestinal permeability induced by cow milk in suckling rats. *Gastroenterology* 1993;105:1643–50.

40. Dugas B, Mercenier A, Lenoir-Wijnkoop I et al. Immunity and probiotics. *Immunol Today* 1999;20:387–90.

41. Neish AS, Gewirtz AT, Zeng H et al. Prokaryotic regulation of epithelial responses by inhibition of IκB-α ubiquitination. *Science* 2000;289:1560–3.

42. Elewaut D, DiDonato JA, Kim JM et al. NF-κB is a central regulator of the intestinal epithelial cell innate immune response induced by infection with enteroinvasive bacteria. *J Immunol* 1999;163:1457–66.

43. Gerwitz AT, Rao AS, Simon PO et al. *Salmonella typhimurium* induces epithelial IL-8 expression via Ca(2+)-mediated activation of the NF-κB pathway. *J Clin Invest* 2000;105:79–92.

44. Steidler L, Hans W, Schotte L et al. Treatment of murine colitis by *Lactococcus lactis* secreting interleukin-10. *Science* 2000;289:1352–5.

45. Shanahan F. Immunology. Therapeutic manipulation of gut flora. *Science* 2000; 289:1311–2.

46. Atlas RM. Probiotics – snake oil for the new millennium? *Environ Microbiol* 1999; 1:375–82.

47. Berg RD. Probiotics, prebiotics or 'conbiotics'? *Trends Microbiol* 1998;6:89–92.

48. Shanahan F. Probiotics: Science or snakeoil? *Clin Perspectives Gastroenterol* 2001: 4:47–50.

49. Konings WN, Kok J, Kuipers OP et al. Lactic acid bacteria: the bugs of the new millennium. *Curr Opin Microbiol* 2000;3:276–82.

50. Shanahan F. Probiotics and inflammatory bowel disease: from fads and fantasy to facts and future. *Br J Nutr* 2002;88(Suppl. 1):S5–9.

51. Rachmilewitz D, Karmeli F, Takabayashi K et al. Immunostimulatory DNA ameliorates experimental and spontaneous murine colitis. *Gastroenterology* 2002;122:1428–41.

Abbreviations

ACCENT	a Crohn's Disease Clinical Trial Evaluating Infliximab in a new Long-term Treatment Regimen
ANA	antinuclear antibodies
ANCA	antineutrophil cytoplasmic antibodies
APC	adenomatous polyposis of the colon
ASCA	anti-*Saccharomyces cerevisiae* antibodies
bid	twice a day
CAM	cellular adhesion molecule
cANCA	cytoplasmic antineutrophil cytoplasmic antibodies
CARD	caspase-recruitment domain
CCR	CC-chemokine receptor
CD	Crohn's disease
CDAI	Crohn's disease activity index
CDR	complementary-determining region
CIR	controlled ileal release
CSF	colony-stimulating factor
CT	computed tomography
DNase	deoxyribonuclease
dsDNA	double-stranded DNA
DZ	dizygotic
EGF	epidermal growth factor
ELISA	enzyme-linked immunosorbent assay
ESR	erythrocyte sedimentation rate
EUS	endoscopic ultrasound
Fc	fragment crystallizable
FDA	Food and Drug Administration

FDG	fluoro-2-deoxy-D-glucose
GAB	goblet cell antibody
G-CSF	granulocyte colony-stimulating factor
GH	growth hormone
GI	gastrointestinal
GM-CSF	granulocyte-macrophage colony-stimulating factor
HACA	human antichimeric antibodies
HCTE	helical computed tomography enteroclysis
hGH	human growth hormone
HLA	human leukocyte antigen
HLA-DR	human leukocyte antigen-D related
I-κB	inhibitor of nuclear factor-κB
IBD	inflammatory bowel disease
IBDQ	inflammatory bowel disease questionnaire
IC	indeterminate colitis
ICAM	intercellular adhesion molecule
IFN	interferon
Ig	immunoglobulin
IIF	indirect immunofluorescence
IL	interleukin
IL-2R	interleukin-2 receptor
IV	intravenous
JNK	c-Jun N-terminal kinase
KGF	keratinocyte growth factor
LPS	lipopolysaccharide
LRR	leucine-rich repeat
MadCAM	mucosal addressin cellular adhesion molecule
MAPK	mitogen-activated protein kinase
MBL	mannose-binding leptin
MHC	major histocompatibility complex
MICA	MHC class I chain-related gene A
MICB	MHC class I chain-related gene B
MLH	MutL homolog
MLS	maximum LOD score
MR	magnetic resonance
MRE	magnetic resonance enteroclysis

MRI	magnetic resonance imaging
MTX	methotrexate
MZ	monozyotic
NBD	nucleotide-binding domain
NF	nuclear factor
NOD	nucleotide-binding oligomerization domain
NPV	negative predictive value
NRAMP	natural resistance-associated macrophage protein
OD	once a day
OR	odds ratio
PAB	pancreatic antibody
pANCA	perinuclear antineutrophil cytoplasmic antibodies
PET	positron emission tomography
PO	by mouth
PPD	purified protein derivative
PPV	positive predictive value
PRE	per rectum enema
rh	recombinant human
RICK	RIP-like interacting CLARP kinase
RR	relative risk
SC	subcutaneous
SCFA	short-chain fatty acid
SNP	single nucleotide polymorphism
TABS	transabdominal bowel sonography
TDT	transmission/disequilibrium test
Th	T-helper
TNF	tumor necrosis factor
TNFR	tumor nerosis factor receptor
Tr	T-regulatory
UC	ulcerative colitis

Index

A

C

D

E

I

Also available from Remedica Publishing . . .

ANAL AND RECTAL DISEASES

Eli Ehrenpreis: University of Chicago, USA

Although rectal and perianal complaints are among the most common seen by primary care physicians, surgeons, and gastroenterologists, the wide variety of disorders associated with these complaints are, in general, poorly understood. Additionally, a variety of newer diagnostic techniques, such as endoscopic ultrasound, mannometry, and magnetic resonance imaging, are now being employed for the evaluation of these disorders. Finally, new pharmacotherapies, including immunosuppressants and topical therapies as well as new surgical treatments, have emerged. This book describes all of these areas in a clear, user-friendly manner.

Contents:
- General information
- Benign anorectal disorders
- Diagnostic procedures
- Neoplasms of the rectum
- Neoplasms of the anus
- Infectious disorders of the anus and rectum
- Miscellaneous conditions
- Patient information

**Available in all good bookshops
and on-line from August 2003**

ISBN: 1 901346 67 6
ISSN: 1472-4138

US$30 / £20 / €30

IMMUNOLOGY FOR GASTROENTEROLOGISTS

Tom MacDonald: University of Southampton School of Medicine, UK

Immunology is a very complicated topic that many people find intimidating. Nonetheless, many gastrointestinal diseases are immunological in origin or exhibit significant immunological components. This book unravels the subject of immunology into three clear areas: immunology itself, gut immunology, and inflammation. Detailed and easy-to-understand explanations of these areas are given, with a focus towards those aspects of immunology that are important at the site of the gut. In addition, this book contains a highly illustrated A to Z listing of over 35 commonly encountered gastroenterological disorders (including: chronic granulomatous disease, Crohn's disease, graft-versus-host-disease, pernicious anemia, refractory sprue, and ulcerative colitis). Detailed descriptions of each disorder cover areas including clinical features, epidemiology, diagnosis, immunopathogenesis, and treatment.

Contents:
- A beginner's guide to immunology
- A beginner's guide to gut immunology
- A beginner's guide to inflammation
- Gastrointestinal diseases with an immunological component
  (over 35 diseases)
- Glossary

**Available in all good bookshops
and on-line from September 2003**

ISBN: 1 901346 56 0

US$30 / £20 / €30

PEDIATRIC GASTROENTEROLOGY AND CLINICAL NUTRITION

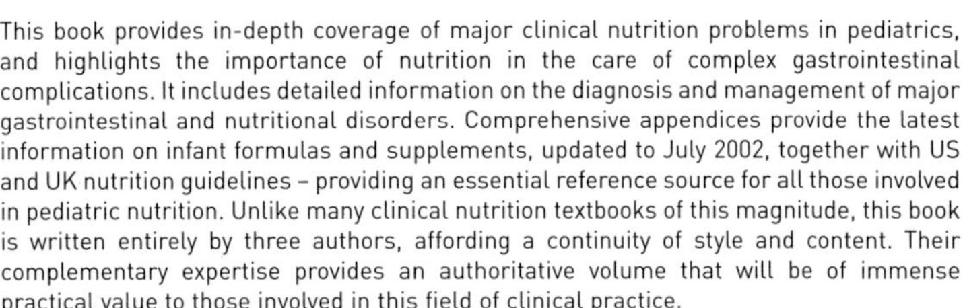

Donald Bentley: Imperial College of Science Technology & Medicine, London, UK

Carlos Lifschitz: Children's Nutritional Research Center, Texas, USA

Margaret Lawson: Institute of Child Health, London, UK

This book provides in-depth coverage of major clinical nutrition problems in pediatrics, and highlights the importance of nutrition in the care of complex gastrointestinal complications. It includes detailed information on the diagnosis and management of major gastrointestinal and nutritional disorders. Comprehensive appendices provide the latest information on infant formulas and supplements, updated to July 2002, together with US and UK nutrition guidelines – providing an essential reference source for all those involved in pediatric nutrition. Unlike many clinical nutrition textbooks of this magnitude, this book is written entirely by three authors, affording a continuity of style and content. Their complementary expertise provides an authoritative volume that will be of immense practical value to those involved in this field of clinical practice.

"This textbook is a valuable reference source for pediatricians, family practice physicians, nutritionists caring for children, and pediatricians-in-training or students with a pediatric interest. It should be strongly considered by any physician or student physician dealing with infants and children for whom nutrition is considered to be an important part of their approach to practice."

Prof Allan Walker, Harvard Medical School, USA

Contents:

- Nutrients and dietary recommendations
- Enteral and parenteral nutrition
- Protein energy malnutrition
- Selected inborn errors of metabolism
- Carbohydrate malabsorption
- Malabsorption syndromes
- Protein-losing enteropathies
- Chronic and recurrent abdominal pain
- Constipation and encopresis
- Inflammatory bowel disease
- Necrotizing enterocolitis and short bowel syndrome
- Gastroesophageal reflux
- Hepatobiliary disease
- Pancreatic exocrine insufficiency
- Eating disorders
- Food intolerance and aversion

Available NOW from all good bookshops and on-line

ISBN: 1 901346 43 9

US$90 / £60 / €90